Communication Skills for Working With Elders

Second Edition

Barbara Bender Dreher, PhD, is Professor Emerita of Communication and former director of the speech and hearing curriculum at Wright State University in Dayton, Ohio. She holds the Certificate of Clinical Competence from the American Speech, Language and Hearing Association and presents many workshops for professionals in health care and human services. She has served on national and state committees on the communication disorders of adults and was a founding member of the Ohio Research Council on Aging. After acting as a consultant with the Greene County Health Department, she founded the first support group for stroke victims in southern Ohio. While serving as a family caregiver she built an extensive record of professional and semi-professional publications.

Communication Skills for Working With Elders

Second Edition

Barbara Bender Dreher, PhD

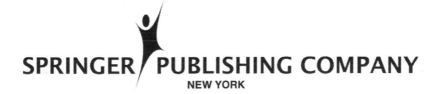

SPRINGER PUBLISHING COMPANY
NEW YORK

Copyright © 2001 by Springer Publishing Company, Inc.

Springer Publishing Company, Inc.
11 West 42nd Street
New York, NY 10036

Cover design by Susan Hauley
Acquisitions Editor: Helvi Gold
Production Editor: Jeanne W. Libby

08 09 10 / 8 7 6

Library of Congress Catologing-in-Publication Data

Dreher, Barabara Bender.
    Communication skills for working with elders / Barabara Bender Dreher.—2nd ed.
      p. cm.
    Includes bibliographical references and index.
    ISBN 0-8261-1405-9
    1. Social work and the aged.   2. Communication in social work.   3. Communicative disorders in old age.   4. Interpersonal communication.   I. Title.
    HV1451.D75 2001
    362.6—dc21   00-067051
                                                                                      CIP

Printed in the United States of America by Berryville Graphics.

Contents

Introduction

The elderly make up the fastest growing segment of our population, and there is increasing national interest in their well-being. The upcoming generation of baby boomers will be choosy consumers—discriminating and demanding. Historically, most resources have gone into meeting the older person's basic needs for health, housing, economic security, and compensatory services. Now there is growing recognition that the served population wants more than satisfaction with bread and butter issues. They want a better quality of life. They want "happiness."

The pursuit of happiness is the birthright of every American, regardless of age. But the full flowering of a personality can be impeded by diminished sensory acuity, muscular strength, and intellectual agility. Professionals are needed to assist the individual in the kind of meaningful activities that maintain integrity, preserve wisdom, and enhance personal relations.

Communication is the key to a happy psychosocial adjustment. It is more than talking and listening, or reading and writing. It is a tool for the kind of social interaction that can aid understanding and overcome loneliness. It is the code for formulating our thoughts and analyzing our emotions. Human happiness depends on the quality of the messages we send to others and the quality of messages we send to ourselves.

The goal of this book is to overcome the barrier of silence often suffered by the elderly and to enhance the quality of their lives. The barriers may be physical—an ill-fitting hearing aid or surgical removal of the vocal cords; social—loss of friends or a restrictive relocation; or emotional—fear of rejection or lowered self-esteem. The professionals who work to remove social and emotional barriers for the elderly are just as vital as those who work to remove physical barriers. Their concerted efforts will help give the elderly that feeling of well-being that comes with improved communication.

The revision of this book involves more than updating research and adding more practical strategies. It addresses new issues like computer use, the characteristics of the "Boomers," the growth of assisted living, the increased need for affordable drug therapies, and new approaches to the depleting emotional strain of anxiety and depression.

Readers will discover how aging itself affects communication as a physical act, and how the expected, gradual changes in the body's tissues, muscles, and nerves affect voice, articulation, and hearing. They will learn how particular illnesses (cancer, stroke, degenerative neurological diseases) can distort speech and language. New tables allow for quick reference to medical conditions and the associated communication disorders. Possible ways to exchange messages despite such physical barriers are included in several chapters.

The social barriers to satisfying communication (changes in residence, dependency, or status) are addressed in chapters on interpersonal and group communication. The section on decision making shows how partial, incremental assistance can give the elderly a sense of autonomy (and resultant cooperativeness) in necessary life choices.

There is a new chapter on computers and the oldest generation. Young people have found that the computer is not just a means for calculating. It is a tool for communication and empowerment. Tapping just a few of its applications can vastly improve the comfort level and self-efficacy of the aged.

The emotional benefits of good communication are discussed in the chapters on promoting self-expression and preserving morale. Making a permanent record of one's life is approached as both an aesthetic and cathartic experience. How elderly persons can vary the quality of messages they send to themselves (as well as the quality of messages they send to others) to increase personal happiness is the topic of the final chapter. Each chapter concludes with exercises and activities designed to help readers practice and increase their skills in communicating with elderly people.

The impetus for this book came from the author's experiences in working for a county home health care agency and in presenting workshops for nursing homes. As a state representative on a federal grant to the American Speech, Language and Hearing Association she became aware of the needs of the non-institutionalized elderly. Ineffective communication behaviors can occur without physical cause and have a depressing effect on the older person and his/her family.

This book offers employees in the health and helping professions practical techniques as well as new methods for enhancing communication with aged clients. As an undergraduate text it will help those who are planning careers that involve the elderly. Communication specialists, speech pathologists, audiologists, nurses, doctors, clergy, physical therapists, occupational therapists, social workers, activity directors, and recreation therapists need communication information and skills to facilitate their earliest internship experiences. Positive communication behaviors will become good habits that will last through years of professional service and yield continuing benefits to the elderly.

1

Bridges to Understanding

The need for special techniques of communicating with children has been accepted for many years, whereas adults are assumed to be able to cope on their own. After all, they have more experience and understanding.

That assumption, however, is not always true. And if and when accommodations are made for the elderly, they are similar to those made for children and are likely to increase dependence and lower self-esteem. What is needed instead are specialized accommodations suited to the broad diversity of the elderly's needs, strengths, and individualities.

Aging in itself is alienating, especially in a youth-oriented society. The pace of technological change is so fast it is readily noticed, but subtle social and cultural changes occur just as continuously and inexorably. We all grow up as creatures of our time, shaped by current events and by our peers. Passage of time places us in various categories with various social expectations. Age alienates—by happenstance more than by calculation. It changes the way we relate to one another and creates the need for special communication techniques to bridge the gap.

Communication should bring people and ideas together. When even the independent elderly, integrated into family and community, experience barriers, how much greater are the barriers for the dependent elderly, enmeshed in various health care facilities? When simply shaping sounds and marshaling vocabulary is a tremendous hurdle, how much more difficult is speaking tactfully and purposefully?

The philosophy of this book is that communication is a two-way interaction. The elderly are not objects, but people, and we do not speak to or at them, but with them. We need to accept their uniqueness as individuals, their feelings, their right to choose and act. Likewise, we need to share our humanness and feelings with them. Because the book is people-centered, many of the problems and solutions are based on real persons whose names are disguised and whose symptoms are generalized. These people typify a growing population.

Bridges to understanding rise from two piers—the fields of communication and gerontology. This chapter will survey the basic theories and phenomena of communication activity and the basic theories and phenomena of aging. Succeeding chapters will build the spans relating the two fields as they reveal the strategies used to meet the needs of real people. Some bridges will rise over the physical barriers; others will span social and emotional gulfs.

Successful communication comes from mutual respect and mutual effort. Young and old, healthy or ill, professional or patient, sender or receiver—we must recognize our common humanity, if there is to be a quality interchange. The reader, with knowledge and willingness, can make it happen.

TWO-WAY NATURE OF COMMUNICATION

Communication is the cohesive force in every human culture and the dominant influence in the personal life of every one of us. As a field of study it uses models to illustrate the process. In fact, there are many models, because a human is not as simple as a machine for which blueprints show all connections. But any graphic representation is a good reminder of the interrelated factors in a communication act. The linear model grew out of years of tradition in public speaking. It looks like this: Speaker-subject-audience-occasion.

It begins with a speaker transmitting a subject to an audience on a particular occasion. The last element answers the questions of where and when, while the previous elements tell who, what, and to whom.

Among the weaknesses of this linear, one-way model were the assumptions that situations were static and that listeners were passive, rather than active, interpreters, responding from their own unique perspectives. Theorists as venerable as Aristotle knew that the speaker was influenced by the reactions of the audience and might alter the message to elicit favorable reactions, but the emphasis of the model was on the first two elements. An authoritative speaker explaining a subject clearly could not fail.

A Case in Point

It was just such a reliance on himself and the information he was supposed to convey that led Chuck into one of the most embarrassing moments in his career. Just three weeks after he started as a social worker in a Senior Outreach program, the police contacted his supervisor with a complaint. A woman had phoned police headquarters accusing him of being a "masher" and of making sexually suggestive remarks to her.

Would a case worker risk his career by harassing a client? Did the police know the woman was 78 years old, living alone? Was this a May-December romance?

The incident developed this way: An agent from Adult Protective Services asked Chuck to manage the case of Ola X, because she was confused about her public benefits. Specifically, "Why isn't Medicare paying my rent? Other women say it pays their rent!" So the two men arranged to see her.

When they arrived Ola seemed friendly. Early conversation went easily when she discovered that she and Chuck shared the same Appalachian background. Then the men got down to business, explaining at length the Outreach service of administering public benefits, the assistance in evaluating current insurance coverage, the disclosure of financial assets and liabilities, and so forth. The other agent was impressed that Chuck had learned the system so quickly. Chuck was proud of that, too, and covered everything very thoroughly. Neither man seemed to notice that Ola said nothing, that the line between her narrowing eyes could indicate suspicion, not concentration. They both urged her to sign the release form. She did. They went away congratulating themselves on a successful interview—until the next day.

Ola's perceptions of the meeting could have been permanently damaging to Chuck's career had there not been a witness. Now when he hears only one voice in a long interview, a red light starts flashing in his head.

The Process Model

Since one-way, top-down communication can lead participants into a corner, it is wiser to think of communication as a two-way process. Then the receiver of the message becomes as important as the sender. The process model is pictured this way:

(Sender—message—channel—receiver)

The sender is the person originating the message idea. The message is the verbal or nonverbal (tone of voice, facial expression) symbolic behavior. The term is general enough to account for the fact that messages may be written as well as oral. The channel is the acoustic, visual, or electronic medium through which the message is transmitted. The receiver is the person or persons listening. These four variables are continuously interacting, and the two end roles can switch back and forth.

Under normal circumstances, the sending and receiving go on simultaneously, and the persons playing those two roles perceive them to be interchangeable. Furthermore, when the message is vocal, the sender's own sound feeds back to him/her and may bring out spontaneous modification in production. When the message is written, a time lapse allows for calculated modifications. The two roles demand skill in encoding, decoding, and interpreting messages.

When people communicate all the factors that characterize them as unique, human beings step into play. These factors are intrapersonal and interpersonal. Intrapersonally, an individual is influenced by heredity, environment, culture, education, vocabulary, life experience, and past communication experiences. Interpersonally, the individual is influenced by the nature of the situation, images of the self as sender/receiver, and images of the other person as sender/receiver.

The equality and democracy implied by two-way communication appeals to everyone. Of more importance to the elderly is the need to participate, to exercise one's rights in the process. Psychologists have noticed that people of advanced age seem to withdraw, to disengage from social contacts. Butler and colleagues (1998) affirm that not all people who live alone are lonely, because isolation may be a habitual lifestyle, not the result of loss. Regardless, involution and depression are assuaged by good interpersonal communication. Relating to other people is both therapeutic and growth-producing. Translators of Martin Buber's philosophy crystallize the idea: "Man becomes man with the other self. He would not be man at all without the I-thou relationship."

FUNCTIONS OF COMMUNICATION

The functions of speech and language are broad and pervasive. This statement is fully understandable when we accept the fact that the ability to communicate is both the essence of humanity and the tool of human interaction. Communication can give all persons a power that is not physical strength. It can help them understand the nature of the world, of other people, of themselves.

The following four functions are adapted from a classification by Dance (1988):

1. To link the individual with his/her milieu or environment
2. To regulate internal and external behavior of others
3. To regulate mental, emotional, and physical behavior of self
4. To develop higher mental processes

If these purposes are interpreted broadly they can cover almost all communication acts. Furthermore, though an act may serve more than one function, this description will help in analyzing the dominant function.

The first function, linking individuals to their environment, can work on several levels. On the rational level it is informative communication that makes direct reference to the physical world. On the social level it is the courteous chit-chat that keeps relationships in good working order. On the emotional level one may talk just to hear oneself, that is, to prove one's existence in a strange or quiet place. A lonely person may talk to a cat or other pet as a way to keep in touch with the immediate environment. Talking to plants or animals is not a sign of age but merely a concomitant of living alone.

The second function of speech and language is to regulate the internal and external behavior of others. Basically, it entails the sending and receiving of messages to facilitate communal life. In the context of controlling social behavior we use rhetoric to persuade others. Politicians and clergy, for example, are concerned with our internal attitudes and beliefs as well as with our outward actions.

The third function is regulating the internal and external behavior of the self. Speech helps us identify and display ourselves to others. Ego demands it. When older people have low self-esteem they avoid meeting new people and hence avoid displaying themselves. If language skills are practiced at a Senior Center or Toastmaster's Club there is a good chance that self-disclosure will not be feared.

Language regulates the person's internal affective reactions by providing a means of expressing and rationalizing emotions. The stroke victim who is deprived of speech is likely to feel choking frustration or blind despair. Language helps to structure life experience into the kind of chunks with which a human being can cope.

Lastly, speech and language help develop the person's higher mental processes. Thinking, in part, is covert or implicit speech. It is not surprising that scientists have found that we engage in subvocal speech during most mental tasks. By measuring muscle movements electrically they found that the tongue and other speech organs were active although the person remained silent. In one experiment, subjects, wired for movement, were asked to imagine counting, to multiply 11 by 99, to recall the national anthem, and to think about infinity. Look up from the page now and try one of these tasks. What are the lyrics of the Star Spangled Banner?

In each of these activities—imagination, recall, concrete and abstract thinking—there was increased activity of the speech muscles.

The speech muscles also make tiny movements when we listen and when we write. In verbal learning tasks such as memorizing words, these muscles are active, although the learner is unconscious of them. In a typical experiment, one group of students was asked to learn a list of words; another group was given the same list, but each subject was told to bite a wooden tongue depressor placed deep enough in the mouth so it inhibited movements of the speech muscles. On a retest the biting group scored much lower than those learners whose muscles were uninhibited (Miller & Johnson-Laird, 1976).

The muscular counterpart of language is not always detected in the speech organs but in whatever muscles express one's interior language. John Singer, the deaf mute hero in Carson McCuller's novel *The Heart Is A Lonely Hunter*, would catch himself moving his hands when he was alone, and he would feel as embarrassed as we would feel if we were caught talking aloud to ourselves. Another study measured hand movements in sleeping deaf subjects. At the onset of dreaming there were increased hand movements showing that language is used in dreaming.

There seems to be overwhelming evidence that language and the ability to think go hand in hand. We admit that putting our ideas into words is an effort. It is an effort because we are coordinating the inputs of imagination, memory, abstract thinking, and critical reasoning. Yet, nudging ourselves to formulate and express ideas is the way to exercise and refine all the contributory mental acts.

The mere effort to communicate helps to maintain alertness. It also prevents egocentrism and disengagement. Because it is a two-way process, it encourages the speaker to see life through the listener's perspective. It may even lead the speaker to be concerned with the code itself. The speaker may try to arrange the message poetically or aesthetically in order to have the greatest impact on the listener.

The various functions of communication are prominent at different stages in life. For instance, the regulation of internal behavior as part of the discovery of self is prominent in late adolescence and young adulthood. Establishing good interpersonal relations takes prominence when increasing helplessness and ill health make the aged person more dependent on others. While it is always therapeutic to release anger through words rather than violence, it is especially valuable to use language when poor health precludes physical expression of emotion.

In general, the elderly have a greater need for good human relations than the middle-aged. They need ties to reality, to family, and to friends to counterbalance the forces of aging. They can achieve good relations by communicating verbally (with tact, clarity, and expression of positive as well as negative feelings) or nonverbally (with smiles, touch, and eye contact). No matter how drastic the barriers, professionals can find compensatory equipment or model attainable behaviors so that the older person can maintain human ties.

NEED AND DESIRE FOR COMMUNICATION AS A VARIABLE OF PERSONALITY

Necessarily, the form and function of communication vary with the basic personality types and age characteristics of the persons involved. Social workers and recreation directors quickly learn the self-concepts of the seniors they work with. Health care professionals are concerned with each patient's self-perception because it indicates coping style. Treatment takes a team and patients who take a share of the responsibility fare better. Self-efficacy entails managing one's health habits, drug compliance, and rehabilitation.

As complex and mysterious as human personality is, major thinkers have defined broad types. These delineations are not based on the stars or the bumps on your head, nor are they highly scientific. But they attempt to answer the basic human need for understanding and predicting behavior by classifying the actor. Certainly, they are preferred to carrying a club as a way to determine whether the strangers you meet on the road of life will treat you with hostility or hospitality.

Carl Jung, the Swiss psychiatrist, first named the two personality types that have had the broadest popular acceptance. They are the introvert and the extrovert. Such archetypes represent ends of a spectrum and no living being fits either category absolutely or exclusively.

Introverts are imaginative, creative, and sensitive. They tend to delay their emotional expression until they analyze the situation and their motives. The subjective world holds high interest for them. They do not seek company but prefer communicating with their own thoughts.

Extroverts, in contrast, are gregarious and prefer communicating with other people. They have high interest in the objective, physical world and take steps to control the environment. An extrovert is a person of affairs—public, political, and practical.

Extrovert Personality

Some mornings when Joseph started to shave he noticed a fine engraving on his cheek. It was the imprint of his watch; he often forgot to take it off before bed. Was he still Time's slave? He did not look like a smooth-faced robot, because his face was too craggy and his skin too pock-marked. He remembered the pirate Captain Hook, in Peter Pan, who was obsessed by the ticking of a clock. Time had ruled Joseph for so many years, he just could not shake it. During his working years, his cohorts were disappointed in his frequent failure to meet deadlines. As engineers they had a fundamental interest in observing and controlling the objective world. Joseph, too, took pleasure in solving down-to-earth mechanical problems, but he also had a terrific yen to be popular. He often spent more time chatting socially, discussing theories, and grousing about workloads than actually working. A former mentor eventually figured out how these opposing characteristics had blended so thoroughly in one person.

Joseph chose his occupation in his late teens, precisely at the time he was experiencing considerable social rejection. The happy-go-lucky boy had been converted into a grumpy misanthrope by severe acne. The eruptions of pus on a face that was already obtuse enraged Joseph and totally frustrated every dermatologist's efforts. Without analyzing himself, Joseph rejected social life and chose a career that required a relatively small amount of personal interaction.

The acne abated only after Joseph's career was established. Then, his natural extroversion came to the foreground. Everyone at the company—from vice-presidents to janitorial workers—knew who he was and what his favorite jokes were. (Joseph loved to tell jokes, and although it took him a tediously long time, the audience always joined him in his obvious relish of the punch line.) He joined recreational clubs and acted as toastmaster for special luncheons. By mid-life he was a moderately heavy drinker who was known for his flamboyant dancing and singing at parties.

Upon retirement Joseph's social interests took on more serious content. He became active in local politics and monitored the Common Pleas Court. He was popular with the other court watchers and developed some accuracy in predicting judgments. Only during the month before an election did he feel social rejection. The young people who volunteered for the campaign avoided him because they thought he was a bit of a buffoon and too talkative to tolerate.

Introvert Personality

Larry was a loner. Like the solitary cowboy riding into the sunset, Larry straddled his motorbike and drove into the desert. His face was tanned as leather and creased with age. He was an active member of the Sierra Club and an avid weekend outdoor-person. Few people would have guessed that his true vocation was law. Most people think of law as a highly verbal profession. But Larry was no talker nor was he gregarious. He had been a solitary child who made friends slowly. At school he was shy, but the girls discovered him because of his green eyes and general good looks. All during high school he restricted himself to casual dating, because for every girl who felt rewarded by his attention, there was another who felt rejected. He tried to analyze his behavior and carried out in his own mind mock trials of The Ladykiller. He criticized himself for getting enjoyment out of the girls' rivalries.

Larry's hobbies as a young man were art and science fiction. He especially liked to draw the rugged landscapes of the Far West as they might be seen through the eyes of a gopher or an eagle. When he tried writing science fiction he also peopled his vision. He tried to show how a person might adjust to an astral environment. The future intrigued him. He wondered how people would cope in the year 2020.

If he had been more practical and more willing to bend his thoughts to suit a consumer, Larry might have made a living as a professional writer. Instead, he turned to law. The long hours of solitary reading and study did not phase him. He steered clear of courtroom exhibitionism and concentrated on theory. He became a professor of law at a major university and was not required to retire. From age 50 on he cut back his working hours to allow more time for his family and his ranch. At age 70 he was still guest lecturing, writing, and editing on his "indoor" days.

Social Impacts

It would also be a mistake to judge concern for others on the basis of personality type. It is tempting to say that introverts only love people at a distance—philosophically. It is equally tempting to say extroverts do not love people as they are but only as a reflection of themselves. True respect for humanity and the ability to get along with people may not be analogous traits. Facile interpretations of behavior as self-serving or public-serving are often wrong. Andrew Carnegie, the extravagant patron of the musical arts, once observed that philanthropy is but enlightened self-interest.

Both the need and the desire for communication are basic to all human personalities. Humans are the social animals, the thinking animals, and only they have the unique physical and mental powers for speech. It is expressive speech (or its graphic representation in writing) that reveals language. No other species comes close to possessing such an elaborate system of arbitrary symbols to represent perceived reality.

Perception of the need and desire to communicate is limited by a person's own definition of communication. In a sample interview, people described communication as "public speaking, memo-writing, propaganda." They rarely mention touching as nonverbal communication or thinking as intrapersonal communication. When the definition is broad the respondent readily admits a tremendous dependence on communication.

FORM OF COMMUNICATION AS A VARIABLE OF PERSONALITY

The forms of communication can be conveniently classified under receptive and expressive types. Receptive forms are listening and reading; expressive forms are talking and writing.

Introverts are likely to be avid readers on topics that suit their mental set. They tend to listen well, too, when they can exercise selectivity. Listening to gossip or chit-chat often will not interest them. But they can be very empathic listeners when a confidante is verbalizing a soul-searching experience. Young people often seek the advice of an older introvert when they are going through personal examination of their goals and values. The introvert has the wisdom not to advise, but to listen, as the speaker explores all avenues and makes personal choices.

Expressively, introverts are likely to prefer writing to speaking. They will shy away from speaking in public. They will not make a toast at the 50th wedding anniversary but may compose a poem for the couple. In writing, they are more likely to keep a diary or journal than to send letters. Their writing is rarely intended for a broad readership or display. The goal is to objectify their own intellectual growth (as in a journal) or to leave a record of historical events and relationships for posterity, as in a family history.

Extroverts are likely to avoid reading as it does not represent immediate reality. They would rather interview someone to gain information about the here and now. They are good listeners, especially for the pauses that indicate that another speaker can have a turn. Their listening span is short, and they prefer the dialogue of TV talk shows to lectures. It is deceptive to see several older extroverts chatting in a group. The "conversation" one expects may actually be simultaneous monologues. The remarks exchanged show no listening to the previous speaker's content but only random comment drawn from one's own mental set. Nevertheless, the participants may feel companionable.

Expressively, extroverts prefer speaking to writing. In fact, experiences in the business world may have made them suspicious of written agreements. They grab for the telephone or make a luncheon date and reach a verbal agreement face to face. (By contrast, the introvert business-person often relies on a written contract.) For absent family and friends long-distance phone calls are preferred to letters. Since extroverts are not reluctant to speak in public, they are often chosen for leadership positions. They work for or against an issue with equal interpersonal skill, and listeners admire their style whether or not they buy the ideas. They are most effective when their reputation for understanding the issue is high and their performing skills do not draw attention to themselves.

THEORIES OF AGING

Knowledge of aging is the second foundation for building a bridge to another generation. Without experience we depend on what society teaches us, and different cultures have different prescriptions for and expectations of the elderly. Social gerontology, the science of aging in society, has spawned several theories to account for the psychosocial changes observed in individuals and groups. Disengagement theory and activity theory are the predominant influences in the field today.

Disengagement theory, first described by Cummings and Henry (1961), explains the social withdrawal observed in many older people. The aged recede socially and psychologically from their environment and relinquish control functions in work, family, and social institutions. This withdrawal is not an imposition by society but an intrinsic result of biological and psychological changes in the individual. The theory is weakened by the fact that there is great individual variance in the amount of withdrawal observed and that those who withdraw do not testify to high satisfaction with the inevitable reduction in interaction.

Activity theory, discussed by Atchley (1994), maintains that substantial levels of physical, mental, and social activity are necessary for successful adjustment to aging. It claims that the amount of social participation is determined by socioeconomic forces and earlier lifestyle rather than by age. There is support for this theory in attitude surveys of the aged; those who reduced their activities expressed reduced overall satisfaction with life.

Recreation therapists, social directors, and most practical workers in the field favor the activity theory. From examining longitudinal data over decades of an adult's life, Atchley (1999) noted continuity in ways of adapting. Humans tend to use well-established habits of mind to make sense out of new conditions and events in their world. Seniors do not stagnate but make flexible changes that follow their customary lifestyle choices. A jogger, for instance, who undergoes hip replacement becomes a walker, rather than a bridge player. Some life transitions present great challenges, but maintaining continuity in the general patterns (not specifics) helps the elder to cope.

No formula for the behavior of the elderly will suit all individuals. Different personalities must be taken into account, for each person is aware of his or her own body changes and social reinforcements. For purposes of discussion, the two major personality types, introvert and extrovert, could be compared for amount of withdrawal and activity. Complex as personality is, it tends to stabilize and intensify over time. Does this fact negate any single theory of aging?

How do the theories of aging affect the need and desire for, and the form of communication? If the elderly are satisfied with withdrawal, they may feel no need or desire for any form of communication. If, on the other hand, their activities were neither reduced nor modified by age, their communication skills would need no reinforcing.

New Aged and Old Aged: Impact of the Baby Boomers

In a democracy, numbers count. A majority vote determines who will lead, what laws will be passed or rescinded, and what policies will guide procedures. How is it possible to balance the needs of 3 million old aged against the wants of 76 million new aged?

In the economic world, too, numbers count. Merchants want a high volume of sales on high-value products, so a population concentration like the Baby Boom has huge influence. If the health care marketplace responds swiftly to the "wants" of the new aged, the 3 million old aged may gain corollary benefits.

When soldiers came home after World War II they wanted to finish their education, find jobs, marry and build families, and buy a house. They had survived the horrors of war by hanging on to a dream and legislators passed the G I Bill of benefits and subsidies to make that dream come true. The Baby Boom generation is the 76 million Americans born in those 19 postwar years 1946–1964. After January 1996 a baby boomer turned 50 years old every 7 1/2 seconds. By 2011 those same boomers will be turning 65 years old at the same rate and straining the retirement system.

Because of sheer numbers this group has virtually recreated American society as it moved through successive life stages. Born into families where the head of household was educated and earned a higher than average salary in an industrial (rather than agricultural) society, boomers had freedom from chores and enough spending money to support retailers of music, clothes, cars, and other goods. With a combination of self-indulgence (the drug culture) and idealism (civil rights) they generated the Youth Revolution of the sixties, the "me" (entitlement) generation of the seventies, and the upwardly mobile set of the eighties. Since they set the trend for each decade in the past, there is every reason to believe they will set trends for the future as they age.

Kenneth Dychtwald (1999), a psychologist and gerontologist, describes the boomers as better educated and more affluent than the oldest generation and predicts their impact on society. They will avoid stereotyped "senior activities" and be drawn to programs that depict their group as healthy and self-confident. They will avoid physical hassles and look for the security offered by corrective and protective products. Advertisers who hope to sell wrinkle removers and hair restorers will tap into vanity, but will find these customers to be choosy. They will use the Internet to get life-enhancing information and will approach purchase decisions rationally. Although they will always be anchored to the cohort values and beliefs of their era, they will also add life-stage roles like mentoring. In maturity they will reject mere accumulation of possessions and will search for products and services that enrich their experience of living.

A large proportion of the boomers have managed their own careers and finances. They have actively maintained their physical and psychological fitness. This tendency toward self-efficacy will continue and they will play an active role in their own health care. Fortuitously, medical science has recently found ways to relieve many age-related conditions like arthritis, prostate enlargement, and menopausal discomforts. With their voting power and affluence boomers will press for more medical breakthroughs. In services they will demand competence; in products they will demand reliability and validity. As educated partners in the health care process they are likely to comply with medications and regimens they help to select.

Boomers will have a big impact on health care. A physician, (Clarfield, 2000), himself a boomer, makes this facetious prediction:

> When my generation of Baby Boomers reaches old age I will be very happy to quit the practice of geriatric medicine. The present cohort of older people is a far more pleasant, patient, less demanding generation. Ours, with its consumerist, demanding, narcissistic nature will be intolerable when it reaches the 7th and 8th decade.

There is a strong contrast between the new aged and the old aged. The old aged are content to start the day with coffee and a donut; boomers prefer to start with a Pepsi or a carrot juice/vitamin cocktail. The majority of the old aged are female and disabled—they comply without asking questions. The new aged exert a healthy ego and question everything.

The fastest growing segment of the U.S. population is the 85 and over age group. Of these, 20% live in nursing homes, and up to 60% are no longer able to manage the basic activities of daily living (Current Population Reports, 1998). Sadly, the incidence of Alzheimer's Disease, a degenerative brain disorder, increases with age. While 4% of the population contract it by age 65, 47% have it by age 85. Step by step the disease destroys the victim and exhausts family caregivers. Duration averages 8–10 years. Conquering Alzheimer's Disease would add "life" to the life span.

Chronic conditions like arthritis, heart disease, and diabetes plague people aged 65 and older. In this age group, 80% have one or more such conditions. Another 50% have two or more ailments, and 25% have problems grave enough to limit daily activities such as bathing and cooking. Laditka (1998) used microsimulation techniques to predict nursing home use under the condition of improved life expectancy. Results showed that better health did not change the proportion of lifetime in nursing homes or the percentage of the cohort who enter nursing homes. However, for the majority of older persons, better health allows more independent living throughout the life span.

CHANGING MENTAL FUNCTIONING OF THE ELDERLY

Mental faculties include such things as drives, motives, emotions, attitudes, knowledge, psychomotor performance, perception, intelligence, sensation, memory, learning, creativity, and the like. While they are all of interest to the gerontologist, only those that most affect one's inclination to communicate will be reviewed at length.

The human mind experiences the outer environment (and the internal, bodily environment) through the senses. With increasing age there can be breakdown of sense organs as well as an increase in the threshold of stimulation needed to activate them. While blindness is rare, many people experience a slow decline of visual acuity, beginning at age 40. The threshold for perception of color and brightness goes up, and driving at night becomes more difficult. The threshold for hearing increases, and sounds must be louder to be perceived. Acuity for high-pitched sounds may become defunct.

The senses of taste, smell, balance, touch, and pain also diminish with age.

Research on perception, the interpretation of sensory data, shows diminishing performance with age. Results are colored by the need for intact sense organs and by the fact that personal testimony is involved. Older subjects are sometimes cautious in stating the presence of a stimulus and rigid in perpetuating their original perception. Inflexibility and the fear of being mistaken grow out of past experience and vary with the individual.

Most central to mental functioning are the complex processes of intelligence and memory. Although biological aging has a definite influence on mental performance, earlier reports that intelligence test scores decline with age are misleading. Cross-sectional studies tested grandparents on skills that were emphasized daily in their grandchildren's school experience. Grandparents scored lower. Such studies failed to equate educational level between the young and the old, and that factor is an important determinant of mental capacity. Longitudinal studies of the same persons over time tend to show stability in measured intelligence (Schaie, 1995).

Because psychomotor performance and response speed decline with age, scores on performance subtests requiring the older person to adduce new relationships yield lower scores than those that test previously acquired knowledge (Botwinick, 1984). Declines are not substantial until past age 70. When they can control the pace of the learning task, oldsters can compete with youthful peers in acquiring new knowledge. They need extra time for both the learning task and the testing of their performance. They do well on tasks that involve manipulation of concrete objects or symbols, unambiguous responses, and low interference with prior learning (Arenberg, Poon, Fozard, Cermak, & Thompson, 1980).

Aristotle recognized memory as "the handmaiden of intelligence," and all tests of memory indirectly test both intelligence and learning. Memory is influenced by attention, by the avenue of sensory input, and by the speed and strength of the original stimulus. For children, the most common memory problem is attention. Hyperactive children are easily distracted by irrelevant stimuli. They can be helped with drugs.

Medical and psychological research indicates that certain organic dysfunctions can contribute to memory impairment. Anemia, arrhythmia (irregularity of the heart beat), thyroid dysfunction, the overconsumption of alcohol, or the use of hallucinogenic drugs are biological factors that contribute to such impairment. Abuse of prescription drugs, such as sleeping pills and tranquilizers, can also result in permanent or temporary memory loss.

Memory is difficult to measure because there can be a breakdown in any of the three stages by which it is developed. First, there is registration or encoding, then retention or storage, and lastly, recall or retrieval. Encoding is an active, even willful process. A person perceives a stimulus, organizes the input, and integrates it with existing knowledge. After a period of time the person is asked to recall the information that was encoded and stored. Elders can compensate for declines by linking new information with their vast store of existing concepts (Perlmutter & Hall, 1992).

Researchers also divide memory into levels (Zek, 1995). Primary or short-term memory covers inputs that will be used or forgotten in minutes. Working memory is the manipulation of information in the short-term base. Secondary or long-term memory stores newly acquired information. Remote memory stores well-learned material and the events of a lifetime. Although all kinds of memory decline with age, there is more loss in secondary memory and working memory.

Intelligent elderly are less susceptible to these losses and so are the people who exercise their memories. Since logical memory declines more than rote-learned memory, repetition is one way to retain inputs. Mnemonic cues help, too. Short-term memory, for example, is reinforced by graphic or verbal rehearsal. Why else are tennis players expected to call out the score and golfers to write down the number of strokes? As age increases, the retention of things heard may be better than the retention of things seen, and the use of both senses together yields better retention than the use of either separately (Arenberg et al., 1980).

For normally aging adults, unfortunately, there is no special vitamin or drug that prevents memory loss. The claims that certain nutrients build brain chemicals are not substantiated. Scientists have discovered special chemicals called neurotransmitters that carry information from one brain cell to another, but so far there are no treatment breakthroughs (Butler, Lewis, & Sunderland, 1998).

SOCIAL EXPECTATIONS AND REALITIES

Because the difficulties of the elderly stem, in part, from the structure and functioning of society, their situation is defined as a social problem. Government acts, like the Social Security Act, which seemed beneficial at the time, had some unpleasant results. By mandating retirement at age 65, with a reduced, but secure, income, social security answered the prayers of the 66% of older Americans who were on relief during the Depression. On the other hand, it stigmatized anyone over age 65 as old, unproductive, incompetent, and expendable.

With rapid social and economic changes, the largesse of the 1940s became inadequate. Inflation diminished the buying power of all retirement incomes, and institutionalized job discrimination prevented individuals from remedying their own money problems. Although Social Security aimed at rewarding the elderly for years of service, it actually removed them from the mainstream of society. Later legislation alleviated these pressures, and both poverty and dependence declined.

"Ageism" is the term coined by Butler, Lewis, and Sunderland (1998) to capsulize the automatic prejudice against the elderly, whether it is caused by resentment of the economic responsibility or fear of the younger person's own death or infirmity. Negative attitudes have made the elderly one of the most neglected and misunderstood groups in our country.

The irony of the ageist system is that society determines and continues to maintain the conditions that allow it to exist. Obsessive fear of death has led to a rise in technologically induced longevity. Average life expectancy has nearly doubled since the turn of the century. Today the average life span is 76 years—up from only 47 in 1900. A full 80% of all deaths occur after age 65. Yet, the World Health Organization reports that there are 23 countries with higher life expectancies than the United States (1998).

Part of ageism is the competition for dollars. The elderly represent 13% of the population now, over 33 million, and the proportion may go up to 20% in the next century if birthrates continue to decline. The average retired couple receives $22,000 a year from Social Security (in addition to any other pension). The figure is regularly and automatically readjusted to cover increases in the cost of living. Younger workers resent the increases in the payroll taxes that make these assured payments to retirees. So legislators raised the original age of retirement. Beginning in 2000 the age 65 limit will go up gradually until it reaches 67 in the year 2027.

Another way in which Congress tried to ease the burden on younger workers was by encouraging the elderly (if able and willing) to continue working. Legislation in 2000 removed the earnings limits on many retirees. Persons aged 65–69 had been penalized if they earned more than $17,000 annually. The Social Security benefit was reduced $1 for every $3 earned. Canceling the penalty is evidence of the new goals and power of the age movement. As elders have grown in numbers and financial security they have influenced politics. The American Association of Retired Person is said to be the largest special interest group in the country (Dychtwald, 2000).

The thrust of the age movement today is to promote autonomy, to pry open possibilities for choice, and to keep them open as long as possible. Elders have the wisdom and desire to leave a legacy for the next generation. To release this potential for bringing about liberating and humanitarian changes, communication will be needed more than ever. In any struggle for progress, all parties to the interaction will need to express, understand, and negotiate with consummate skill.

Reality Check: Health Care and Prescription Drug Expense

When Medicare began in 1965 the government spent about $100 per year for the average old person. By 1995 the cost had risen to $7000 per person. Currently the elderly account for 44% of all hospital-bed days and 24% of physician office visits (National Center for Health Statistics, 1995). They run up additional costs, averaging $2750 annually, which are paid out-of-pocket. This includes supplemental insurance premiums, co-payments, deductibles, and prescription drugs.

By the end of the 1990s prescription drug prices had grown to a crisis level. Average out-of-pocket expenses for the one-third of Medicare's noninstitutionalized beneficiaries who had no drug coverage was just under $600 per year (Gross & Brangan, 1999). Worse still, many were paying ever-rising premiums for private supplemental insurance that covered other medical gaps, but not prescriptions. Some individuals felt pressured to choose between food and medicine, to ration their pills or their meals. While they were likely to have lower incomes than beneficiaries with drug coverage, they were not poor enough for Medicaid. Eligibility for state Medicaid programs measures value of assets as well as income, so a widow living in her own home might not qualify.

The situation had evolved out of Medicare's need to avoid costly hospitalization and nursing home costs. Drug therapy and home care seemed to be a solution. So doctors prescribed more drugs, and drug companies expanded research to develop remedies for more ailments of the aged. Prices for the 50 drugs most used by seniors increased faster than the rate of inflation, causing hardship to the 35% of all Medicare recipients who had no other coverage.

Inadvertently, the government itself contributed to the high price of new drugs by patent requirements for both safety and efficacy. Exclusive patents last just 6 years and then generic versions are allowed. Herbal remedies and food supplements are not held to such high standards. Further, legitimate drug companies may face product recalls and lawsuits from individuals or groups. These entail legal expenses whether or not compensation must be paid.

Currently drugs cost more in the United States than in Mexico, Canada, and Europe. Pharmaceutical companies point to differences in exchange rates, standards of living, and likelihood of product liability law suits. Some governments control prices or profits. Pressure groups want the United States to do the same even though profits fuel innovation. Inevitably, the federal government will play a role in containing costs for the drugs seniors need (Getz, 2000).

EXERCISES

1. Watch prime time television for one hour, and write down the ages of all persons who appear on the screen. Make separate lists for the featured shows and the advertisements. How many people over age 65 appeared in the show? In the advertisements? How were they depicted?

2. Make a list of 10 adjectives that describe these two common stereotypes: 1. the wise old man; 2. the dirty old man.

3. Complete the Communication Activities Survey (Table 1.1) by interviewing a family member or acquaintance who is over age 65. How do you account for the high or low rankings on particular items? Personality? Environmental influences? Or

TABLE 1.1   Communication Activities Survey

	Low	Medium	High
1. About how many hours would you say you watch TV on a day like yesterday? ( ) hr	2 hr or less	2–5 hr	5 or more hr
2. About how many hours would you say you listened to the radio yesterday? ( ) hr	Less than 1 hr	1–2 hr	2 or more hr
3. About how many hours would you say you read yesterday? ( ) hr	Less than 1 hr	1–3 hr	3 or more hr
4. How often do you visit with your neighbors in the building (in town)? (verbatim answer)	Less than daily	Daily	More than daily
5. All in all, how often do you see any of your friends and relatives in town? (verbatim answer)	Monthly or less	Monthly to weekly	More than once a week
6. Do you recall how many phone calls you made and received yesterday? ( ) calls in: ( ) calls out	2 or fewer calls	3–4 calls	5 or more calls
7. How often do you go to church?	Never	Sometimes	Weekly or more
8. Do you belong to any clubs, civic groups, or voluntary organizations? Which ones?	None	1	2 or more
9. How often do you attend meetings of these groups? Weekly, monthly, less often? (verbatim answer)	Never	On irregular basis	Regularly

Adapted for Graney, M. J., & Graney, E. (1974). "Communication Activity Substitutions in Aging," *Journal of Communication, 24*(4), 88–95.

partial employment? The division into high, moderate, and low activity categories was originally based on 92 response sheets from women (median age 75.3 years) in a metropolitan housing development.

REFERENCES

Arenberg, D., Poon, L., Fozard, J., Cermak, L., & Thompson, L. (Eds.). (1980). *New directions in memory and aging.* Hillsdale, NJ: Lawrence Erlbaum Associates.

Atchley, R. C. (1994). *The social forces in later life: An introduction to social gerontology* (7th ed.). Belmont, CA: Wadsworth.

Atchley, R. C. (1999). *Continuity and adaptation in aging.* Baltimore, MD: Johns Hopkins University Press.

Botwinick, J. (1984). *Aging and behavior* (3rd ed.). New York: Springer.

Butler, R., Lewis, M., & Sunderland, T. (1998). *Aging and mental health* (5th ed.). Boston, MA: Allyn & Bacon.

Clarfield, M. (2000). Baby boomers then and now. *Geriatrics and Aging, 3*(3), 38.

Cummings, E., & Henry, W. (1961). *Growing old.* New York: Basic Books.

Current Population Reports (1998). Washington, DC: U.S. Bureau of the Census. Author.

Dance, F. E. (1988). Introduction to communication. In C. Carmichael, C. Botan, & R. Hawkins (Eds.), *Human communication and the aging process.* Prospect Heights, IL: Waveland Press.

Dychtwald, K. (1999). *Healthy aging: Challenges and solutions.* Gaithersburg, MD: Aspen.

Dychtwald, K. (2000). *Age power.* New York: Jeremy Tarcher/Putnam.

Getz, A. (2000, July 10). In defense of prescription drug prices. *Newsweek,* p. 3.

Gross, D., & Brangan, N. (1999). *Medicare beneficiaries and prescription drug coverage: Gaps and barriers.* Washington, DC: AARP Public Policy Institute.

Laditka, S. (1998). Modeling lifetime nursing home use under assumptions of better health. *Journals of Gerontology, Series B: Psychological Sciences and Social Sciences, 4,* 177–187.

Miller, G., & Johnson-Laird, P. (1976). *Language and perception.* Cambridge, MA: Belknap Press of Harvard University Press.

National Center for Health Statistics (1995). Health, United States, 1996–97. Washington, DC: Author.

Perlmutter, M., & Hall, E. (1992). *Adult development and aging* (2nd ed.). New York: Wiley.

Schaie, K. W. (1995). *Intellectual development in adulthood: The Seattle longitudinal study.* New York: Cambridge University Press.

World Health Organization (1998). *The world health report 1998: Life in the 21st century—a vision for all.* Geneva, Switzerland: Author.

Zek, R. (1995). The neuropsychology of aging. *Exp. Gerontol., 30,* 431–442.

2

How Aging Affects Communication

SOCIAL CHANGES THAT AFFECT COMMUNICATION

In addition to the dominant theories in the social psychological study of aging—disengagement and activity, there is a newer approach—ecological systems. It emphasizes that the environment either provides or withdraws opportunities and means for authentic social interactions. Children move away, and the costs of transportation and telephone may reduce communication. Friends, siblings, and spouses may die, and the depth of social interactions is reduced to shallow niceties. Moving to a new community with a better climate may deprive the oldster of the uninhibited, but all-accepting, interchanges with familiar neighbors.

While the major social change that affects communicative interactions of the elderly is loss of family or friends either through death or separation, society intervenes only when institutionalization is required. Roughly 5% of the elderly cannot take care of themselves and need nursing home care. The changes in residence and personal relationships destroy old communication patterns.

There is no conscious attempt by social and health care agencies to curtail communication opportunities, but necessary protection of one segment of an older person's life may inadvertently cause deprivation in another segment. For instance, the communications systems in nursing centers that measure physiological functioning of the body or signal distress, fire, or emergency tend to dehumanize the environment. The patient does not need to speak when objective clinical tests are considered more reliable than personal testimony. The person begins to feel like a guinea pig or an object. Such a situation results in a decrease in the informative and social functions of oral communication.

Dependent Living

Although poor health necessitates the institutionalization of almost 2 million elders currently, by 2030 that number is expected to double. Affluent baby boomers who have worked consistently on a healthy lifestyle will live longer than their ancestors did. But eventually they will experience debilities which require comprehensive professional care, including the services of communication specialists. Long-term-care residents trade off individuality to gain security and continual health care. Personal freedom is constrained by medicine and diet schedules, the use of prosthetic devices, and the activity and mobility limits imposed by disease. The emotional results can be devastating.

Fear arises first because the situation is unfamiliar. The fear of pain, of death, of desertion, all compound to block out any communication input. When the fear is joined by anger, the patient drifts into self-pity. The anger is projected onto family members and makes them feel guilty.

When the family members fail to understand the older person's need to vent feelings and receive negative messages at face value, they are tempted to avoid further meetings. Listening to complaints, justified or not, is unpleasant. A decline in visits then reinforces the patient's fear of being deserted, and isolation is compounded with desolation.

Interpersonal communication with the family or old friends is rarely compensated for by ties to the other nursing home residents. Roommates are assigned not chosen. Residents may have widely different interests and backgrounds—ethnic, socioeconomic, and religious. Each patient feels he/she is different, singular, and alone. At first one may not bother to develop confidantes, because the stay is hoped to be temporary. Later, the patient often becomes too discerning of the differences in the other people and fails to recognize their common humanity.

Neither does the patient strike up personal relationships with the staff. They are seen as givers of service, not as individuals. Communication is used to make demands, to complain, and to parry superficial social observations. Messages from the physician or the administrators are rare and may be poorly understood because of the patient's declining memory or impatience with detail. Daily communications with lower level staff and other residents may be inaccurate and tainted with rumors and projected fears, thus contributing to the patient's overall anxiety.

Long-term care is the most regulated industry in the United States (Chop & Robnett, 1999). Due to media exposure and complaints from families and consumer groups, legislators passed a reform package as part of the Omnibus Budget Reconciliation Act (OBRA) in 1987. This act led to a greater emphasis on staff training, regular in-service programs, and resident rights (including rights to dignity and privacy). It instituted systematic assessment of the resident's mental and physical health (minimum data set) upon admission and at regular intervals thereafter (Bonifazi, 1998).

OBRA requires a safe and homelike setting. Recreation therapists aim to maintain each individual's functional capabilities and to promote quality of life. Other therapies flourished in the 1990s—mental health, speech-language, occupational, and physical. In 1998 Medicare set annual payment caps for such services, while still recognizing that therapy prevents patient decline. Another cost-cutting policy at that time was requiring electronic transmission of patient care records. Nevertheless, all states now have ombudsmen to protect nursing home residents and to advocate for wise policies.

To enliven the monotony of institutional life, long-term homes have added birds, cats, and dogs to the environment. They have added courtyards, gardens, sun-rooms, and plants. They make space for children, families, and entertainers of all kinds.

One of the most idealistic and comprehensive movements is the Eden Alternative (Thomas, 1996). Beginning in 1991 in a single facility in upstate New York, it had spread to 200 homes by the turn of the century. It featured the environmental changes mentioned above plus self-governing care teams that work consistently with the same group of residents. Like a family, chores are shared and even residents assume some responsibility. Staff children, school children, or on-site day care centers counter the boredom, loneliness, and helplessness of institutional life.

Even with donations and volunteers, there are added costs (like obedience training for the dogs), but the life-focus in the workplace seems to lift the morale of staff, too. There is less burnout.

The Eden Alternative claims that creating a human habitat will dramatically reduce the number of medications that residents require. Other administrators warn that it takes a complete shift of mindset for physicians and staff to resist prescribing (Halbert, 2000). Nevertheless, when patients feel happily involved they are less likely to complain, balk, wander, or withdraw.

Another growing trend in long-term care is the provision of *Special Care Units* for people with dementia. The National Institute on Aging (1996) reports that more than 15% of nursing homes have added Alzheimer wings. These units are safe, but not restrictive. Residents may stroll freely from the dining area to a sun porch to an enclosed yard with circular paths, even though a coded security system prevents them from wandering away from the establishment. Facilities are designed to be bright and homelike (one assisted living community advertises a "special neighborhood for the memory-impaired"). Rooms have lots of light to eliminate frightening shadows and help reduce depression. Light is especially needed in the late afternoon when Alzheimer patients become agitated ("sundown syndrome"). They ask to "go home," but the home they mean refers to the favorite place of childhood. While craft activities are still popular, the newest facilities have kitchens and laundry rooms where residents can wash dishes and fold clothes. Doing adult tasks gives them a sense of accomplishment and dignity (Kalb, 2000). Staff members relinquish some of the controlling behaviors needed in acute care. Instead they try to understand the patient's world. The National Institute on Aging reports that special care units help patients maintain physical functioning and positive behaviors. Both the setting and the philosophy of care have improved residents' quality of life as evidenced by increased social behavior and interactions (1996).

Continuing Care Retirement Communities

A hassle-free place to live and health care for life can be obtained at continuing care retirement communities (CCRC's). The homes vary from freestanding housing to condominiums and apartments of varying size and opulence, to private hospital rooms, as needs change. Originally this choice was only available to the rich, because of high entrance fees and monthly fees. There is a wide range of services for the setting—housecleaning, yard upkeep, transportation—and for the individual—meals, laundry, rehabilitation, medication management, nursing care, and social and recreational programs. Daily life can be enjoyable until illness strikes or chronic conditions exacerbate. Then the individual is guaranteed space in a nursing facility while the spouse or other family member can continue to live independently. To become more affordable some CCRC's now offer modified contracts with specified levels of long-term care. Even more modest is a fee-for-service plan whereby the resident pays separately for whatever services are needed.

Assisted Living

Since the 1980s assisted living has become an important category in the continuum of care between total independence and round-the-clock medical support in a nursing facility. Patterned after Scandinavian systems, this living arrangement allows the frail elderly to age with dignity. Residents are not treated as patients, but as social, spiritual individuals. Ninety percent of these facilities are paid for with private funds and every effort is made to provide social stimulation and courteous, effective communication. The services, activities, and employee training are customer-centered and include the caregiving families. Because of the founding philosophy and the staff training communication problems are few.

There is no single definition of assisted living. To avoid federal regulation, providers have chosen to work with state agencies to self-define standards, measurement, and monitoring. Most of the largest providers are publicly held and managed as for-profit businesses. Many states are trying to include low-income seniors through waivers to the federal Medicaid program because this housing is less expensive than 24-hour care in a nursing facility.

American Demographics reports that nearly half of people aged 85 and older require some assistance with at least one activity of daily living (ADL), such as bathing, dressing, and getting in and out of a chair or bed. Additionally, they need help with some Instrumental Activities of Daily Living (IADL), such as meal preparation, shopping, taking medications properly, paying bills, or using the telephone (Barton, 1999). These services are paid for as needed and are not part of the rent.

The 85 plus population grew at a rate of 39% during the 1990s and is expected to grow at 33% in the next decade. Assisted living complexes are increasing at 15 to 20% per year (Weaver, 2000). Caregiving families may be entering the ranks of the young-old and need this type of placement for their parents. As the trend grows there is increasing competition. To reach full occupancy some complexes may add residents with increasing dementia and/or medical needs. A fair contract spells out under what circumstances a resident would be required to change rooms or move out of the facility altogether.

Shared Households

Communication barriers are different in both kind and quantity for the almost 20% of older Americans living with their children and grandchildren (Clark & Niedert, 1992). Two- and three-generation families living in the same house tend to have problems in deciding who is dominant. Because of tradition, the oldest man in the household expects to exert authority over both the middle-aged parents and the grandchildren. However, many believe that the leadership belongs more appropriately to the person whom society holds responsible economically. While the whole family should engage in discussion, final decisions remain with the responsible person.

By relinquishing their authority, grandparents often gain a new feeling of freedom. They can relate to their adult children as friends and to their grandchildren as allies in a subdominant position. In fact, alternate generations often find more ideas in common as social values swing from one world view to the next. The "back to basics" movement as manifested in the educators' return to the 3 R's and the popularity of natural foods and nontechnological methods of homemaking has drawn the elderly and young adults together.

Group living, whether with family or nonrelated adults, requires communication to regulate the internal and external behavior of others. Coercive or rejecting messages must be replaced with appealing and reconciling messages. Words and acts of consideration help everyone to maintain self-esteem. Family counselors should be called in when deep conflicts occur over the division of labor, responsibilities, or privileges.

Independent Living

Communication patterns are least distorted for the older person who lives independently at home. About one-third of these independent elderly are widowed, divorced, or separated. About one-half of all women older than 65 are widows (Bureau of the Census, 1998). So a typical situation is a widow trying to manage the house where she lived as a wife and mother for most of her existence.

Married couples living independently seem to have all the advantages for healthful, happy aging, but there can be drawbacks. They may have limited communication because of rigid adherence to former role assignments and work habits. They may neglect making long-range financial and health care plans by clinging to the vague hope that death will come quickly and painlessly in the night. Whoever dominates in the pair may avoid sharing authority through fear, selfishness, or short-sightedness.

The single person living alone feels no threats to autonomy in the activities of daily living, but there may be loneliness or lack of stimulation in the home environment. Although there is less communication input without a daily companion, there can be enjoyment of television, radio, newspapers, books, letters, telephone calls, and visits. Chat rooms or support groups on the Internet can be stimulating, too. The better the person's health, the more social contacts can be maintained in the community and the extended family. Illness and/or incapacity are very real fears.

If the residence has too many stairs, too much noise, poor insulation, poor access to transportation, and requires too much maintenance, an elderly person may move into an apartment or condominium especially designed for the elderly.

It is likely that a loner will avoid relocating because of finances, resistance to change, or fear of the unknown. Nevertheless, neighbors, family, or community services such as Telephone Reassurance perform a real service when they make a daily contact with this aged person. Autonomy is further strengthened by communicating wishes for the future to the responsible next of kin.

PHYSICAL CHANGES THAT AFFECT COMMUNICATION

Typically, advanced age can make a person's voice tremulous, weak, hoarse, and higher or lower pitched than it was in middle-age. The elderly may testify: "I can't sing the way I used to," "If I talk too much I have to clear my throat a lot," or "My voice tires quickly, and I get hoarse."

Listeners notice the difference, too. Just by hearing they can determine the age and sex of an unseen speaker. It is a judgment most frequently made when answering the telephone or listening to the radio. What is amazing is the accuracy with which these judgments are made. Although such symptoms are bothersome, they are considered a normal consequence of aging, particularly after any structural abnormality, vocal abuse (smoking), or pathology has been ruled out. Joel Kahane (Kahane & Beckford, 1991) made a long series of studies of the aging speech mechanism, so professionals could pick out the few differences that signal pathology. He found decreased mobility of the overall laryngeal structures, decreased efficiency of muscle contraction, and reduced range of motion at laryngeal joints. Nerves going to and from the larynx degenerate, too.

Changes in Articulating

Articulation is the process of shaping the vocal tone into significant oral symbols. It requires various muscular adjustments. Vowels are formed by the tongue and lips taking particular positions while the airstream passes freely out through the mouth. The consonants require more adjustments of the jaw, lips, tongue, and soft palate as the airstream is blocked, squeezed, or forced through various channels.

Precision of movement is a key element in the process of articulation. Evidence exists from the studies on perception of age in recorded speech samples that imprecise consonants and slow articulation rate are common among the older speakers. Hence, coordination and speed seem to deteriorate in the speech act, just as in other psychomotor tasks.

Other effects of aging may contribute to small detriments in articulation. Receding gums, poorly fitted dentures, and partial plates can leave tiny spaces and make sounds slushy or whistling. Hearing loss, affecting high-pitched sounds like sibilants, or making voiceless sounds like *p*, *f*, and *t* inaudible, causes trouble. The sounds that are no longer clearly received become neglected in speech production also.

The bad news that hearing loss leads to articulation imprecision is balanced by good news. Hard-of-hearing people tend to talk louder. Since they hear themselves as poorly as they receive other voices, they compensate by putting more energy and intensity into vocal production. This phenomenon aids intelligibility, which depends on loudness as well as articulatory accuracy. Furthermore, speech and hearing clinics give "speech insurance" lessons. Motivated oldsters can learn to monitor their own speech by concentrating on the touch, pressure, and muscle cues of each movement, rather than on hearing themselves.

Changes in Phonation, Pitch, and Timing

Phonation is the process of vibrating the tensed muscular bands (vocal cords) by forcing air from the lungs between them. The bands are located in the center of the larynx (Adam's apple). They are wide open for silent breathing, partly open for whispering, and closely approximated for speech. With increasing age the laryngeal cartilages tend to stiffen and calcify, and the small muscles lose strength and elasticity. Voice samples of older people show a lack of sustained laryngeal tension and air wastage (the vocal folds act as a valve controlling expiratory airflow).

Laryngeal muscles are responsible for the pitch (highness or lowness of tone) of a voice. One's dominant pitch is measured as a fundamental frequency. Lifetime changes in pitch are common knowledge, and Shakespeare reviewed them in his Seven Ages of Man, from the "mewling" infant, to the childhood shrillness of both boys and girls, to the distinct differences between men and women in their sexually active years, to the final similarities in old age. Male fundamental frequency increases progressively from ages 50 to 89, resulting in increasingly higher pitched voices. Elderly women show no consistent changes in pitch, although many report lowered pitch (Weismer & Liss, 1991). So the poet's description holds, and the scientist supports it with evidence that male vocal pitch makes the big changes—both in puberty, as a result of rapid anatomic growth, and in old age.

Voice tremor is a characteristic of the older voice that actors routinely adopt when trying to portray old age authentically. It is an exaggeration of vibrato—the quality that is highly prized by operatic singers. Vibrato is a tremulous effect obtained by rapidly alternating the original tone with a slight variation in the pitch. It adds richness and texture. With biological aging the vocal folds lose resilience and elasticity. The pitch variations around the intended tone get too wide, and vocal clarity is blurred. Kahane and Beckford (1991) called this "jitter" and attribute it to a decreased number of mucus glands and increased viscosity of vocal fold tissue.

Although the opera singer's career is curtailed by reduced breath capacity and decreased control of the expiratory airflow, such respiratory changes do not affect speaking. The speech act requires only medium lung capacity, and air supply can be replenished during normally occurring pauses. Casual singing can be enjoyed throughout life, and the presence of tremor is no cause for worry. Unfortunately, the tremors that accompany neurological diseases, such as Parkinson's, are slower and wider than the normal ones. The broad tremor and slower rate demand more careful listening by others.

Timing in speech refers to both overall speed and rhythm. Several studies have found that elderly subjects have a significantly reduced rate of oral reading. But such a task is affected by many variables including vision, education, and familiarity with the material. Studies of impromptu speech also noted slower rate, but not that much slower. Impromptu speaking is complicated by the fact that it involves memory and the neurological processing of an original message.

A symptom similar to stuttering can be observed in the speech of some elderly people. It seems to be a neurological dysfluency characterized by word repetitions, interjections, and fillers. It lacks the heavy psychological overlay of fear, tension, anxiety, and avoidance that accompanies such behavior in younger people who consider themselves to be abnormal speakers. These "uncertainty behaviors" in the elderly represent the longer times needed to retrieve and associate words. Considering the changes in mental functioning, such nonfluencies should not be considered abnormal.

DELICATE BALANCE IN VOICE AND ARTICULATION

In summation, normal speech requires both energy and relaxation (Figure 2.1). The brain commands graded movements and the ear monitors the result when all systems are healthy. For some old people it is difficult to produce signals that are loud enough, clear enough, and well-spaced enough for a listener to grasp. Weakness, paralysis, poor hearing, or brain damage destroy the delicate balance, and the listener, in turn, must exert the extra effort to close the circle of communication.

CHANGES IN HEARING

Hearing loss begins in the second decade of life and proceeds very gradually with age. Some people are more susceptible to damage than others, and long exposure to industrial noise may account for the fact that after age 55 incidence studies show more men having hearing loss than women.

Just how many of the elderly suffer from presbycusis (age-related deterioration in hearing)? The National Council on the Aging (1999) reports that 9 million Americans over the age of 65 have hearing loss. For the elderly residing in nursing homes and other institutions, incidence figures are wide-ranging because of varying test criteria. Generally, 60% to 90% of the institutionalized elderly experience difficulty in hearing speech.

ENERGY
In skeletal muscles to support posture
In abdominal and breathing muscles to support loudness
In tongue, jaw, lips, and palate to support intelligibility

RELAXATION
In shoulder muscles to support best pitch
In throat muscles to support clear tone
In vocal tract muscles to support best resonance

FIGURE 2.1 Balancing energy and relaxation.

As with the other senses, age affects both the acuity (accuracy of perception) and threshold (minimum amount of stimulation needed to excite a sense organ). Acuity declines because of degeneration of nerve cells and other structures in the inner ear. Hence, older people lose the ability to hear sounds of certain frequencies (pitches). Loss of high-pitched sounds is usually more severe than loss of low-pitched sounds, so the perception of speech becomes a difficult chore. Each person has a unique pattern of loss and the newest digital hearing aids can be calibrated to reinforce only the weak areas. The added clarity comes at a high cost (up to $3000), though, and most insurance policies do not cover it.

The increasing threshold for intensity (loudness) is easier to remedy. Hearing aids can amplify a stimulus until it is loud enough to be heard. After screening by an otologist to determine if there is any reversible medical cause, the person who suffers hearing loss should be evaluated by an audiologist. If an aid is required, several brands should be tried before any is purchased. Using the aid takes repeated practice, and the period of adjustment is about 6 months. Tips on the care of hearing aids are included at the end of this chapter.

The amount of handicap caused by a loss depends on the individual's capacity for social interaction and for compensation visually, by "reading lips." Actually, a variety of nonverbal cues—facial expression, eye lines, gesture—are observed in the speech-reading process. Learning traditional sign language is usually not an appropriate compensation for hearing loss in older persons, because family, cohorts, and social contacts cannot respond to that language (unless they learn it, too).

Recently a complex electronic device has been developed to help the profoundly deaf. A cochlear implant is surgically placed under the skin behind the ear. It scans the environment for useful sounds and sends them to the brain. Cochlear implants can electrically stimulate dead or damaged nerve cells, but, so far, they help primarily the profoundly deaf who get minimal help from hearing aids. The 24-channel implant is intended to enhance speech recognition by delivering more high frequency tones. The process is expensive and there is the standard risk as in any kind of surgery. While reception of environmental sounds improves, speech sounds are still difficult to decipher. The National Institute on Deafness and Other Communication Disorders' Fact Sheet (2000) also cautions that learning to interpret the sounds transmitted takes time and practice.

Hearing and listening should not be confused. It is not always easy for family and friends to distinguish an actual hearing loss from lapses in listening. The former is a physical problem, and the latter is a psychological problem. The persons addressed may be inattentive, uninterested, preoccupied, unwilling to cooperate, or depressed. They do not want to hear.

It is wise to observe behavior when the persons want to hear. If they show signs of strain (leaning forward, cocked ear), ask for clarification frequently, make a constant visual scan of the speaker's face, or complain of dizziness or tinnitus (buzzing or ringing head noises), a hearing assessment should be made. An audiometric exam is an accurate physical measure of the ears' response to sound.

Untreated hearing loss has negative consequences. Without that window to the world, existence is less secure and sociable. In a 1997 study (Resnick, Fries, & Vergrugge) of nursing home residents both moderate and severe hearing loss resulted in less time spent in social engagement and activities. The NCOA study of 2300 hearing impaired persons and 2000 family and friends showed similar patterns. Further, denial of the problem was common. Only 2 of every 5 who needed amplification actually used a hearing aid.

Case Study of Hearing Impairment

While he was still actively employed as a supervisor in the engineering offices of a national manufacturer, Howard was bothered about his hearing. It was not his ears he worried about. It was those fat envelopes addressed to him personally: "Are you troubled by your hearing in the office, at business meetings, at cocktail parties? _____ Co. offers a complete line of hearing aids, in all the latest styles, with all the desired features."

Who was giving his name to hearing aid dealers? Was it one of the younger men at the office who was eager to have Howard's position? Some of those bright guys with MBAs made him feel nervous. In some ways, he wanted to be like them. He bought a van but neglected to shroud it in curtains and murals. (His van looked like an airport bus.) But he drove it as fast as a sportscar!

And who did not have trouble hearing in the office? The typewriters, telephones, and business machines made so much background noise. At meetings some people mumbled; they did not have gumption enough to state their opinions clearly. As for cocktail parties, everyone knows alcohol depresses the ability to hear and to articulate.

What made Howard so angry about these letters was that he was aware of changes in his ability to hear in all kinds of environments. But was it really serious? He has never had medical problems with his ears or throat. It was his brother who had tonsils and adenoids removed at age 50 but continued to suffer from sinus drainage. Howard decided that if he ever felt pain or sickness he would take action, otherwise he would ignore the issue.

Several years after retirement Howard was an official delegate to a church conference. He noticed that the Master of Ceremonies was wearing a hearing aid, and everyone laughed at his jokes though Howard could not quite catch the key words. Returning to his home city, he made an appointment with an otologist who, in turn, arranged to have an audiologist test Howard's response to pure tones and to speech.

The tests revealed that Howard had presbycusis—a reduction in both loudness and clarity of sounds due to degeneration of inner ear structures. Presbycusis usually occurs in both ears. As Howard expected, the otologist found no medical complications and suggested that Howard try a variety of hearing aids by visiting several dealers. Because his wife had come to the office with him, Howard gave up the temptation to ignore the issue. He would not become one of the 6 million Americans who could benefit from an aid but neglect to purchase or use one.

Luckily, Howard's wife made the visits with him and kept a list of the kinds, capabilities, limitations, trial periods, insurance facts, and costs of the various hearing aids on the market. He had trouble enough to keep his senses alert and notice the fine differences in amplification capabilities. He was disappointed to learn that no affordable aid amplified selectively . . . if it made speech louder, it made background noise louder, too. And he knew that the distortion of particular sounds was due to nonreversible nerve degeneration. Other things being equal, he would have preferred an aid built into a pair of glasses, so people would not notice it. However, shrewd shopping and common sense led him to choose a "behind-the-ear" aid. It gave him the best fidelity. Furthermore, he was pleased that the ear mold was custom-made for him and felt comfortable.

Howard might well have used his aid a few times and then left it in a drawer. But a friend at church was enrolled in speech-reading classes at the local speech and hearing center and drove by to take Howard to class. The therapist was gracious and the group members were friendly so Howard joined. He learned what good use he had been making of his eyes as his hearing was deteriorating. By watching lips, eyes, facial expression, and the speaker's whole aspect, he could grasp messages. He learned how to make maximum use of his residual hearing and how to "stage-manage" his environment for better listening.

In a few months, Howard was as accustomed to using his hearing aid as he was to using his reading glasses. The former required a little more maintenance—changing batteries, cleaning wax from the mold—but they were no real problem. And his wife reminded him to have periodic checks for both his eyes and ears, so he could be assured of the best sensory input possible.

The following tables (Tables 2.1 and 2.2) give practical tips for hearing aid problems and for communicating with the hearing impaired.

EXERCISES

To Intervene or Not to Intervene: A Role Play

Instructions: As three students represent these roles the rest of the class tries to determine whether or not there is a bona fide hearing problem. List all the clues that indicate an actual physical loss. List all the clues that indicate a psychological problem (i.e., a listening problem) due to inattention, fear, pride, unwillingness, and so forth. What are the extenuating circumstances and attitudes?

Role players should present the following three scenes:

Scene 1: Betty is telling Jason she has made an appointment with an otologist and why. He reacts.

TABLE 2.1   Emergency First Aid for Hearing Aids

If the hearing aid does not work at all:

   Try a fresh battery, and be sure the "T" contact of the battery matches the "T" contact in the aid.

   Check tubing to make sure it is not twisted or bent.

   Check switch to be sure it is on M (Mike), not T (Telephone).

   Try a spare cord on a body aid. The old one may be broken or shorted.

   Check earmold to be sure it is not plugged with wax. Try a fresh battery.

If sound from the aid is weaker than usual:

   Check tubing for bends and earmold for wax or dirt.

   If aid has been exposed to extreme cold, it may not work until it is at room temperature.

   You may have excessive wax in your ear. See your doctor. *If aid goes on and off or sounds scratchy:* Work the switches and dials back and forth. Sometimes lint or dust will interfere with electrical contacts.

   On body aids, try changing cords. *If aid whistles continuously:* You may need a new earmold or new tubing. See your audiologist.

Scene 2: Betty is complaining to John and they compare observations.

Scene 3: John is checking out Jason's impressions and making a final recommendation.

Characters

Jason Senior: You are an 85-year-old man who lives alone in an apartment. You enjoy your life there. Age has slowed you down a bit, but you still feel quite capable of taking care of yourself. You have several friends in the building and you even like the times you are completely alone so that you can pursue your hobby, photography.

Recently your daughter, Betty Senior Bates, who lives on the other side of town, has been badgering you about a hearing test. You know there's nothing wrong with your hearing. She just mumbles a lot because she's always got a cigarette in her mouth. You feel that she treats you as if you're old and feeble and can't do anything for yourself.

Betty Senior Bates: You are a 55-year-old woman with a family and a part-time job as a secretary for an insurance company. Your mother passed away several years ago, and your father lives alone in an

TABLE 2.2 Ten Tips for Effective Communication with Hard-of-hearing Persons

---

1. Stand at a distance of 3 to 6 feet.
2. Arrange to have light on your face, not behind you.
3. Position yourself within the visual level of the listener.
4. Speak at a natural rate, unless you see signs of incomprehension.
5. Speak slightly louder than normal. Do not shout.
6. Always face the hearing-impaired person, and let your facial expression reflect your meaning.
7. Use short sentences.
8. Rephrase misunderstood sentences.
9. Do not talk while eating, chewing gum, clenching a pipe, or laughing.
10. Identify the topic of conversation so the listener has some contextual clues.

---

apartment on the other side of town. You are very concerned about him living by himself and trying to manage his own affairs independently. He is quite old and just doesn't understand today's world.

He doesn't seem to listen when you try to advise him—he doesn't always hear the phone when you call. You are becoming convinced he has a hearing problem. After you made an appointment with an otologist, you arranged to drive him there. When you got to the apartment he had gone out with a friend.

John Doe: At 66 you are working for the County Commission on Aging as a senior aide. You have been visiting Mr. Senior for the past 6 months. He is an elderly gentleman, but seems to get around all right and has control of his mental faculties. He has done for himself all his life and is offended at the thought of being cared for by someone else. You haven't noticed a hearing problem. You've watched him startle when an ambulance passes in the street. You find Mr. Senior to be forgetful and lonely . . . typical of your clients. That accounts for the one-way conversation.

Mrs. Bates has asked you to resolve their controversy about a hearing exam. Mr. Senior is offended at the thought of being bossed. He is proud of his longevity and good health habits. What can you do?

REFERENCES

Barton, J. (1999). Assisted living: the growing trend in senior housing. *Mature Living, 42*(4), 10.

Bonifazi, W. (1998). Progress in patient care. *Contemporary Long Term Care, 24,* 53–58.

Chop, W., & Robnett, R. (1999). *Gerontology for the health care professional.* Philadelphia, PA: F. A. Davis.

Clarke, C., & Niedert, R. (1992). Living arrangements of the elderly: An examination of differences according to ancestry and generation. *Gerontologist, 32,* 796–803.

Halbert, R. (2000). Focus on care-giving: Lessons from the original 'Eden'. *Provider,* June 2000, pp. 49–51.

Kalb, C. (2000, January 31). Coping with the darkness. *Newsweek, 135*(5), 52–54.

Kahane, J., & Beckford, N. (1991) The aging larynx and voice. In D. Ripich (Ed.), *Handbook of geriatric communication disorders* (pp. 165–180). Austin, TX: Pro-Ed.

National Council on the Aging (1999). *The consequences of untreated hearing loss in older persons.* Washington, DC: Seniors Research Group. Available at: *http://www.ncoa.org/news/hearing/01_intro.htm.* [2000, June 8].

National Institute on Aging (1996). *Progress report on Alzheimer's Disease* (NIH Pub No. 96-1137). Silver Spring, MD: Author.

National Institute on Deafness and Other Communication Disorders (2000, March). *Fact Sheet: Cochlear Implants* (NIH Pub No. 00-4798). Bethesda, MD: Author.

Resnik, H., Fries, B., & Vergrugge, L. (1997). Windows to their world: The effect of sensory impairments on social engagement and activity time in nursing home residents. *Journals of Gerontology, Series B: Psychological Sciences and Social Sciences, 52*(3), 135–144.

Thomas, W. (1996). *Life worth living: The Eden Alternative in action.* Acton, MA: Vander Wyk & Burnham.

Weaver, P. (2000). Assisted living takes off with U.S. support. *AARP Bulletin, 41*(2), 10–12.

Weismer, G., & Liss, J. (1991). Speech motor control and aging. In D. Ripich (Ed.), *Handbook of geriatric communication disorders* (pp. 205–227). Austin, TX: Pro-Ed.

3

Interacting With the Elderly

In face-to-face interactions with the elderly, we send and receive a myriad of verbal and nonverbal messages. Typically, the brain responds to the mass of cues by matching to old patterns or creating new, simplifying configurations. Many of the old patterns are stereotypes passed along by the culture and not experienced directly. The "dirty old man" stereotype from movies and books keeps many a young businesswoman from seeking the advice and help of an older businessman. Likewise, a young intern is dismayed to witness a gray-haired woman swearing like a trooper. Whether a stereotype idealizes or discredits a group of people, it can mislead because it fails to account for individual differences.

Perception is basic to interaction. It is an individual's interpretation of events seen, heard, or otherwise received through the senses. How unique human beings behave in a communication situation depends on their perception of self and others.

HOW THE ELDERLY PERCEIVE THEMSELVES

Self-perception has been categorized in various ways, but the most basic components first appeared in the Tennessee Self-Concept Scale (Fitts, 1972):

1. physical self
2. moral-ethical self

3. personal self
4. family self
5. social self

In rating themselves, even the healthy elderly are generally dissatis-fied with their physical self. Witness the sales of everything from wigs, dyes, and hair-restorers to foot powders and podiatry services. They regret the loss of muscular strength and flexibility. Further-more, they lose reliable input from the eyes and ears, as well as from the other senses. If they fail to acknowledge the wrinkles and sagging flesh in their own mirrors, they see such changes in their cohorts (age mates, often with a shared history). The view of the physical self is even worse for the elderly ill and disabled.

The moral-ethical disposition of the elderly often comes from an earlier era and thus seems dissonant to current lifestyles. Moral standards that were taught and reinforced when they were growing up have become habits that color their perception of present social ways. It is no wonder that stereotypes of the moralizing old patriarch and the frigid old maid abound in popular literature. The fact that younger people tend to avoid those who hand out negative judg-ments leads to further disengagement and loneliness for the elderly.

Age also diminishes the personal self. When your memory plays tricks on you, when your strength does not hold out until a task is finished, when loss of loved ones makes you depressed, and when accumulated petty frustrations make you irritable, it is hard to main-tain self-esteem. Writing from his own aging experience, Skinner (with Vaughan, 1983) notes that the aged blame themselves for the decrements in their lifestyle and, consequently, lose respect for themselves. (Skinner, in contrast, indicts the cultural and social environment.)

In terms of the family, the aged person usually experiences loss of power and increasing dependency. When living with the children becomes necessary, there can be a distasteful reversal of roles, that is, the children taking on the responsibilities and privileges of parents. Increasingly, there are four-generation families where a frail, elderly parent is dependent on an adult child for care, at the same time as this adult child is providing care for grandchildren. Over 100 such "generationally inverse" families were studied by Foulke (1980), and although most of the caregivers were in their 50s, 20% were in their

60s. About 10% of the aged had experienced some form of aggression or threats from the caregiving child. Yet 71% of the aged (especially those short of money, prestige, and mobility) admitted using psychological manipulation to get their way in return.

How do the elderly perceive their social self? Much the way the rest of society does—negatively. Respect for elders, even to the point of ancestor worship, was characteristic of Eastern cultures, not Western cultures. In the United States, modern transportation, industrialization, and mandatory retirement have caused a progressive decline in the status and social integration of the aged. Until 1900, life expectancy was less than 50 years, and there was no sophisticated, life-sustaining medical technology. Without many examples, even the "young-old" (55 to 75) do not have a clear social prescription for "old-old" (75 to 95) behavior. That vacuum is filled by cultural myths and stereotypes presented in the mass media.

Images From the Mass Media

The mass media have erred in both directions by presenting disproportionately positive or disproportionately negative views. Newspapers tend to do personality profiles of elderly people who have unusually creative hobbies or other successes. How many 70-year-old women win the Betty Crocker Award, publish a novel, run a Marathon, or act in commercials? The one-dimensional feature story can be so upbeat that it actually demoralizes the majority of oldsters.

Television, on the other hand, has presented notoriously negative stereotypes. Oldsters were rarely allowed on screen except as victims of crime or disease—boorish foils or hapless fools. At best, the characters were lovable, yet always laughable. In commercials older actors are used to sell laxatives, skin moisturizers, hair dye, and even prescription medicines. Yet it is just this commercialism that promises better treatment for the elderly in the future.

The media respond to market pressures. Our culture is more money-oriented than youth-oriented, and economic recessions gild the value of Social Security income, which, though small, is steady and predictable. Television advertisers have become more aware of the enormous buying power of the growing elderly population. Thanks to Medicare, improved pensions, and Social Security, less than 10% of the aged live below the poverty line. For the young-old, fixed expenses tend to decline as children grow up and become financially independent. In 1998 statistics showed that households headed by someone over age 50 held more than half of all discretionary income in the United States (U.S. Bureau of the Census, 1998). Because of inheritance taxes and changing savings habits, many oldsters use that discretionary income to buy services and products peddled by mass media.

The elderly, like the very young, are often more influenced by the images presented on television, because they have so many hours available for viewing. Repeated exposure strengthens the stimulus. Forty million retirees average 43 hours per week in front of the tube (Media Dynamics, 1999). By contrast, the young career person finds his/her self-concept in the working world. Those elders who have a positive and realistic self-concept tend to behave in healthy, constructive, and effective ways:

> Such persons are more secure, confident and self-respecting; they have less to prove to others; they are less threatened by difficult tasks and situations; they relate to and work with others more comfortably and effectively, and their perceptions of the world are less likely to be distorted. (Fitts, 1972, p. iii)

Such persons develop the self-efficacy health professionals prize because it promotes compliance and self-care. Elders with the capacity to act productively are valuable members of the health care team.

INITIATING AND MAINTAINING RELATIONSHIPS

When a realistic view of oneself includes age, illness, and pain, there is not much energy to bring to an encounter. The person with the healthier self-concept usually takes responsibility for communicating and tries to understand the other person by observing objective properties, social behavior, and unique characteristics. Appearance can range from the overstuffed dowager decked out in jewels and furs to the institutionalized great-grandmother whose nervous hands keep pulling on wispy hair. Social behavior refers to what people say and how they say it. It is sad that brooding old people often reject friendly overtures when they most need them. The unique characteristics refer to the personality, temperament, talents, energy, past activities, and details of life of that particular person.

First impressions of the elderly, especially the institutionalized elderly, can be intimidating to beginners in the helping and health professions. There is a self-protective urge to keep a distance from people with germs, but what conditions the elderly have are not contagious. Any signs of repugnance only make them feel less attractive, so the professionals need self-control. They need the courage to bridge physical, social, economic, and cultural gulfs, as well as the generation gap. If they have grown up with the presence of a grandparent nearby, they have an experience against which to measure a new endeavor. A student nurse shared her experiences and changing perceptions of her grandmother this way:

> In my family I always knew where I stood with my grandparents—that is, until recently. Now I find that the older I get, the younger they seem. As a kid, I loved them but I was a little afraid of them. They'd give me ice cream, but they'd yell if I spilled it on the carpet or deliberately stirred it into mush.
>
> Two years ago things really changed. My Grandpa died, and I got my driver's license. Since Grandma doesn't drive, my family assigned me as chauffeur. So I take her to doctors' offices and for groceries and such. Naturally, our conversations broadened from polite requests about my grades to more personal matters. She doesn't mind hearing about my boyfriend, and she tells me things about Granddad I never expected to hear. When I get angry with my Mom, Gram hears me out.
>
> Exactly how much our relationship changed I didn't realize until all those doctors' visits confirmed bone cancer. Even if radiation works, I know now that she will die someday. It would be easier to face if she were still the feared matriarch, but now I'm going to lose a close confidante.

This student certainly helped her grandmother to survive bereavement and may yet help to prolong her life. Such a close relationship is crucial to the "will to live."

A number of studies suggest that being happy in old age depends on having a confidante, a close, trusted friend to whom one confides intimate meanings—fears, dreams, plans, disappointments. Whereas women choose a confidante among women or men, men almost always choose the spouse. Perhaps this fact can be accounted for by the observation that men get together for specific activities—sports, cards—rather than talk, or that they fear "losing face" before their colleagues in a competitive career world. Regardless, the loss of a spouse as a partner for communicative intimacies can be devastating.

Older persons tend to choose friends from the same community and socioeconomic level. In times of crisis friends provide transportation, care during illness, and comfort during bereavement. Long-term friends can supercede family ties. Research over the past two decades has shown that friends are more important to the psychological well-being of the elderly than family members (Adams & Bliezner, 1995).

In every new interaction, there is an element of risk, because egos can be diminished or enhanced. Younger persons wonder if they will be corrected, advised, or negatively evaluated by the standards of a different era. Older persons wonder if they will be treated as competent or incompetent. When they seek social or health services they are afraid they will be bossed, patronized, or treated like children. Some oldsters seem paranoid, because they have strong memories of trust being violated. Others, who have hearing problems or a foreign language background, seem suspicious, because they may not understand fully what is said to them. Yet, a basic trust in people in general allows almost everyone to move beyond reluctance and to find the rewards of interaction.

The Greek philosopher, Plato, wrote, "The person who knows only his [or her] own generation remains forever a child." More modern philosophers add, "In order to see, you have to be willing to be seen"—reinforcing the principle of self-disclosure. Since revealing information about yourself is the typical introduction you should tell the oldster who you are and where you come from. If similar information is not given in return, ask for it, and ask how the person prefers to be addressed.

Two-way communication means both parties give time, energy, personal information, and some level of emotional support. The parties do not hide behind generalities but make remarks that are specific and concrete. Depending on amount of contact and degree of mutuality, various levels of self-disclosure may be attained. Low-level disclosure is the way most interactions begin—with ritualized greetings, simple inquiries, and comments about the weather or surroundings.

Middle-level disclosure deals with events, hobbies, sports, travel, holidays, and such. Some personal values and opinions are shared. At this level old persons can get beyond their current physical selves and tell about their past experience and accomplishments. Asking them "how to do something" within their scope (former business, cooking, gardening, car repair, etc.) can draw them out, as having advice solicited raises the sense of competency. Roommates in nursing homes often fail to reach this level and never gain the self-esteem that comes from sharing. Free choice and mutual interests may not be considered in placing residents. Furthermore, residents may consider the situation to be temporary and ration their emotional energy for other demands.

When a high level of intimacy is reached, both parties have confidence enough to speak of their personal problems, successes, and failures. They share judgments about mutual acquaintances, trusting that the comments will go no further. The nursing student above had reached a high level of self-disclosure with her grandmother. The emotional rewards were great. Few interactions go so far, although the popularity of psychological counseling services show there is great need. In social situations, good taste, sensitivity to the other party's responses, and appropriateness determine the level of intimacy.

INTERVIEWING

When oldsters seek health and human services the interview is more than an exchange of information, a filling in of blanks on a standardized form. Both participants send and interpret verbal and nonverbal stimuli. Both may lapse into role-playing—the interviewer becomes a "know-it-all" or "keeper of the golden key," and the interviewee becomes "genteel old lady" or "strong, silent hero."

Here are some tips for developing a good interviewing style:

1. Arrange the environment for quiet, privacy, neatness, and comfort. A good setting helps you establish rapport.
2. Keep a box of tissues handy in case people cry. Reassure them that emotional release is acceptable, and wait quietly, perhaps patting a hand or shoulder.

3. Make clear the purpose of the interview, and explain why you take notes or tape record or call in a colleague, if you do.
4. Avoid falling into a mechanical pattern of short answer and "yes/no" questions.
5. Ask open-ended questions that allow for amplification. For example, "How did you make friends?" and "What activities increase the pain?"
6. Use terminology within the realm of the informant. Be alert for nonverbal signs of incomprehension—squinting, furrowed brow, blank or quizzical eyes.
7. If a spouse, adult child, or other caring person has come with the informant, look for patterns of dominance and submission. Informants should be encouraged to speak for themselves if at all possible. The interviewer should focus questions and eye contact in that direction and respond less to the domineering partner.
8. An overly verbal respondent whose content rambles may require a tactful interruption. You can ask for clarification, summarize, or ask a new question.
9. The reticent interviewee can be encouraged with brief remarks ("Tell me more"), nonverbal nods, and brief but attentive silences. Sometimes it may be necessary to rephrase or repeat the question.
10. Use summary and repetition of key points in closing the interview. Ask for feedback to check understanding of what transpired. Thank them for giving time, attention, and cooperation in the process.

INTERACTING EMPATHICALLY

A totally businesslike interview seldom elicits more than "yes/no" responses. Interviewees go away as frustrated as students who face a fill-in-the-blanks test knowing many more answers than fit the small pigeonholes. Not only can important information be missed, but so is the opportunity to build the kind of rapport and trust necessary for compliance later on. Some oldsters continue with quacks and charlatans whose treatments are not effective simply because they are so charming, comforting, and complimentary.

Displaying empathy, the sharing of another's perceptual field and world of meaning, can improve the quality of information exchange. Skilled communicators have to make a conscious effort to neutralize the tendency to interpret another's meaning from within their own internal system of values and perceptions. They can help troubled speakers express their own fears, problems, needs, angers, and expectations.

Communicating partners who have reached a high level of self-disclosure also use empathy. In times of crisis they serve as psychiatric aides for each other—venting feelings, offering support, exploring options, and sometimes planning actions. They can identify with each other emotionally.

Basic to an empathic exchange is respect. The distressed person needs to believe that the listener really wants to understand and will maintain privacy, withhold judgment, and reserve advice for the ripe moment. There is a great deal of literature on empathic listening, but since interactions are two-way it is important to be aware of empathic responding. Comments should be brief, concrete, direct, and jargon-free. Tone and inflections should promote sharing and be fully congruent with body language. Saying, "Of course, I'm concerned," in an angry way, while thumbing through a stack of papers, presents too many interpretations and squelches sharing. Asking for clarification and checking perceptions are good moves. Perhaps the best responses are reflective—a simple reiteration or rephrasing of the speaker's current emotions, perceptions, and plans. Respect for people includes faith that, given time, they can find solutions for themselves.

Oldsters often give advice and resent receiving it (perhaps they perceive it as another diminution of their power and status). Anyway, the empathic process allows them to vent feelings, remember options, and develop insight into situations they may or may not be able to handle by themselves.

Certain responses are definitely not respectful and turn off sharing:

- Minimizing: "It isn't as bad as all that."
- Personalizing: "You think you've got a problem, listen to mine."
- Temporizing: "You'll feel better about it tomorrow."

- Sympathizing: "I'm just as disgusted as you, but what good is that? "
- Universalizing: "Everybody gets discouraged at that."
- Judging: "You really messed up."
- Dumping: "You thought you had trouble. What about those you offended?"

Temporizing can be especially annoying to the elderly. As one old man quipped, "Don't say I've got time. How do you know? I don't. I even hesitate to buy green bananas!"

Feedback

In communicating with the elderly, there are special pitfalls in assessing impact. Neither the longed-for positive feedback (agreement, questions, and volunteering information and opinions) nor negative feedback (correcting, fault-finding, and disagreement) may occur when expected. Many of the elderly simply delay responses; they seem to be inattentive. Actually, they may be trying to match the incoming message with a wealth of data from past experiences.

Not only is feedback delayed, but its nonverbal expression can be distorted by health problems. There is less facial expression when people are tired or depressed (and fully 20% of those labeled "senile" are actually suffering from depression). Certain drugs also inhibit signs of alert listening. A national survey showed that hospitalized Medicare patients receive an average of 9 prescription drugs, including digitalis, diuretics, anti-hypertensives, sedatives, hypnotics, painkillers, and laxatives (Carlson, 1996). Four out of five independent elderly persons have at least one chronic illness for which they receive medication, and which they may complicate by additional over-the-counter drugs. A change in communication style might well be a clue to more serious adverse drug reactions (ADR's).

Oldsters with dementia can interrupt a speaker with "off the wall" comments or try to draw attention by bizarre actions. People recovering from stroke can shake their heads "yes" and say "no" at precisely the same time. They can be moved to tears or laughter without much cause. The person with Parkinson's disease rarely smiles or blinks, yet his/her mind can be fully engaged with the message.

Examples of distorted feedback from the ill and disabled are innumerable, so speakers have to be as gentle in their judgments of their own performance as they are of the listener's. Later attitude changes or behavior improvements may be credited to a particular interaction, or the cumulative effect of several interactions that seemed futile at the time.

GAINING COMPLIANCE

Health care professionals feel frustrated when patients ignore their instructions based on a careful diagnosis and assessment. Intentional or not, noncompliance is wasteful and dangerous. Common types of noncooperation include misusing of medication, not following exercise or diet programs, and engaging in prohibited activities such as smoking or drinking. Research shows that compliance with a medical regimen is about 50% (Salzman, 1995). When taking prescribed medicines 1/3 of patients followed the instructions properly, 1/3 did so "sometimes," and 1/3 did so "almost never."

Assisted living residents often have sensory, memory, or cognitive impairments that interfere with a complex drug regimen. Those living in nursing homes don't even try to self-manage because of confusions with timing, dose power, dose form, and conflicts with already prescribed medications. The frailty of the elderly ill requires professionals to fine-tune dosage levels and avoid overmedicating.

The majority of older patients in the community are not too uneducated or forgetful to comply, but they manufacture their own, fairly logical, excuses. If the symptoms go away, or if the treatment is too complex and stretched over too long a period of time, or if the activities are merely preventive, they are less likely to cooperate. Older persons have a long memory and years of experience with a variety of doctors and medicines and levels of discomfort. Previous doctors may have destroyed their faith in the system. Their judgments and resulting cooperation are affected by their cultural as well as historical background. Those who do worry about their health sometimes think they know better than current health workers.

Whatever the reasons, health care professionals develop persuasive powers to assure cooperation. Patients with whom they have had the longest relationship and have shared the most personal information are usually the most compliant. Because patients have to bare so much of themselves to doctors, they expect some mutuality in return. Trust comes from self-disclosure. The professional's self-disclosure is not just a recital of superior knowledge, but an extension of personal warmth and empathic listening.

Physicians who have had communication skills training score high on teaching patients (Communication skills boost educational outcomes, 2000). Participants at a recent workshop developed these guidelines for gaining cooperation:

1. Establish the need for a medication, action, or prohibition by explaining test results.
2. Check for emotionality. The time to *talk* about test results is not when the person is highly stressed or in pain. If a family member or friend has come to act as advocate, explain to them, too.
3. Check for understanding at each stage by asking questions.
4. Explain what the professional can do and what the patient can do. This step includes monitoring jargon and level of detail to suit the patient's attention span, sensory deficits, and need/desire to know. It means going over written materials that patients take home to review at their own pace. Never assume they will be read.
5. Explain the specific treatment and how other, similar persons adapted to it. Visualize the drawbacks—potential discomfort, possible side effects, and their likelihood of occurrence. Visualize the benefits and the timetable for experiencing them.
6. Set a follow-up pattern of visits and/or phone calls, and/or e-mails so both partners can take remedial action or feel satisfaction in the healing process.
7. Avoid threatening or scaring patients. If a prognosis is too terrifying, listeners repress and try to forget. If the threats do not materialize, all the rest of the doctor's advice is discounted. Exaggerations violate respect and ruin the relationship.
8. Be persuasive but not pushy, personable but not patronizing, and collaborative but not coercive.

EXERCISES

1.   Here are some situations and remarks that could occur when working with the elderly. As a measure of your sensitivity, you are to judge which responses promote or inhibit sharing.

Task 1: Identify the responses that tend to show respect and those that do not. You are not trying to select the best of all possible responses. You are dealing only with respect and nonrespect.

1.   *Recreation Assistant to Director of Senior Volunteers:* "I feel like a ping pong ball. Anybody and everybody tells me what to do. I don't think anybody around here has a clue about what I'm supposed to do."
     a.   You shouldn't let these things upset you so much. They aren't really all that important. After all, it's just a job. It's not your 'whole life.'
     b.   You have to learn to take this sort of thing. Just make up your mind that nobody gives a darn about you around here and forget it.
     c.   You feel like it's open season on you and anybody can tell you what to do.
     d.   You've got a good thing going for you, you know. Talk like that will just get you fired.
     e.   Are you sure that you're not overreacting?

2.   *One Resident of a Retirement Community to Another:* "This is the biggest gossip factory I've ever seen. Everybody's just waiting around to spread some darn lie about you. I'm really fed up with this kind of junk. I want to live some place where everybody isn't out to get you."
     a.   How about yourself? Don't you talk about other people? Sounds to me like you're doing the very same thing right now.
     b.   You shouldn't pay any attention to what other people say. They can't hurt you. Just ignore them. People who gossip are stupid anyway.
     c.   I've felt that way at times. I've wanted in the worst way to zipper some lips—permanently.

     d. I don't care where you go, you'll find the same thing. People like to talk. The only way to protect yourself is try to be as friendly as you can with everybody.

3. *Nursing Aide to Co-Worker:* "I think that the head nurse has just got it in for me. I don't do anything worse than you do or anybody else around here, but when I do the least little thing she really blows up."
   a. Maybe you just think that you don't do anything worse than the rest of us.
   b. Everybody has times when they don't get along with superiors. What's happening to you has happened to everyone at some time or another.
   c. I'm sure that you won't worry about this so much tomorrow. Things will look a lot better to you after you've had time to cool off a bit.
   d. It seems to you that you're being blamed unfairly and you're pretty mad about it.

4. *Community Relations Director to Vice President of Patient Care Services:* "That trainee you assigned me is really bad news. She won't take any directions. Before she knows how we do things or why, she's already giving me advice. Who does she think she is anyway?"
   a. Look, your job is to train her and not get into some stupid personality clash.
   b. Come on now, you're not the easiest person to work for. Maybe you're only assuming she knows what you expect. If I know you, you're probably being pretty unrealistic.
   c. Sounds like she's giving you some real heartburn.
   d. Give her time. She's probably just working overtime to make a good impression.
   e. I know how interested you are in our trainee program. Tell me some more about what's going on.

Task II: Now identify the other responses. Which are helpful, judgmental, minimizing, temporizing, personalizing, sympathizing, universalizing, or dumping.

Other Exercises

1. Set up a two-person communication situation and have one partner tell his/her personal feelings about a news item. The other partner must paraphrase the first message before going on to express his/her personal opinion. A third person acts as observer and recorder. The goal is to evaluate how accurately the partners paraphrase each other.

2. Here are some items from the Philadelphia Geriatric Center (PGC) Morale Scale. With no intention of scoring, use them to guide the content of your conversation with an older person. Your opener can be "How do you feel?"; then stick to that subject for awhile. Listen for the respondent's position on these items without asking directly.

PGC Morale Scale

\# 2 I have as much pep as I did last year.

\# 8 I sometimes worry so much that I can't sleep.

\#15 I get mad more than I used to.

\#18 I take things hard.

\#20 My health is (the same, better, or worse) than most people my age.

\#21 I get upset easily.

3. Set up a dyadic (two-person) interaction to develop empathic listening skills. Let one person role-play the social worker and the other, an aged person. Let the latter describe the events leading up to placement in a nursing home. The social worker should elicit the oldster's feelings about those events.

4. Self-disclosure is part of developing a two-way communication with an elderly person. Write a 100-word paragraph identifying yourself before your first encounter.

5. Perform the following role-play for your classmates. What is the mother's image of herself? What is the son's image of himself? Cross out the lines that block emotional flow; add some lines to make the interchange more positive.

SUNDAY VISIT

Son: How are you doing this week?

Mom: Don't ask (shrugging her shoulders). You wouldn't want to know.

Son: Sure I would. What's the matter?

Mom: Never mind. How are Sally and the kids?

Son: Fine. Now, tell me what's the matter.

Mom: I'll tell you what's the matter. You don't love me, that's what's the matter. You never call. You hardly ever visit. I was so lonesome Tuesday and you never called.

Son: That's my bowling night.

Mom: That's what I mean. Your family comes last! Bowling and clubs and fancy cars. That's all you think about! I could be sick and you wouldn't . . .

Son: (interrupting) If I didn't care about you I'd be out bowling again tonight.

Mom: Go ahead! Forget those who sacrificed for you.

Son: I'm fed up. You never appreciate anything. Goodbye.

REFERENCES

Adams, R., & Bliezner, R. (1995). Aging well with friends and family. *American Behavioral Scientist, 39*(2), 109–221.

Arcangelo, V., & O'Connor, T. (1994). Compliance in the elderly: What factors contribute to medication misuse. *Pharmacy Times, 21,* 30–42.

Carlson, J. (1996). Perils of polypharmacy: 10 steps to prudent prescribing. *Geriatrics, 51,* 26–50.

Communication skills boost educational outcomes: physicians get primer on teaching patients (2000 March). Editorial. *Patient Education Management, 7*(3), 31–36.

Current Population Reports. (1998). Washington, DC: U.S. Bureau of the Census. Author.

Fitts, W. H. (1972). The self-concept and performance. Research Monograph #5. Nashville, TN: The Dede Wallace Center.

Foulke, S. R. (1980). Caring for the parental generation: An analysis of family resources and support. Unpublished Master's Thesis, University of Delaware, Newark, DE.

Media Dynamics. (1999). *TVdimensions '99.* New York: Author.

Salzman, C. (1995). Medication compliance in the elderly. *Journal of Clinical Psychiatry, 56*(1), 18–23.

Skinner, B. F., & Vaughan, M. E. (1983). *Enjoy old age: A program of self-management.* New York: W. W. Norton.

U.S. Bureau of the Census. (1998). *Consumer Expenditure Survey* (1998). Washington, DC: U.S. Government Printing Office.

4

How Illness Affects Communication Skills

Communication disorders constitute the nation's number one handicapping disability. Studies indicate that more people suffer from hearing, speech, and language impairment than from heart disease, venereal disease, paralysis, epilepsy, blindness, cerebral palsy, tuberculosis, muscular dystrophy, and multiple sclerosis combined (ASHA, 1999). While 1 out of 20 people in the United States has a disorder, the number of friends and families affected by reduced communicative interaction is even greater.

Although hearing loss is the most common communication disorder in the geriatric population, there are also speech and language problems caused by a variety of physical traumas. Stroke, cancer, degenerative neurological diseases, and accidents can rob a person of the ability to understand or use the language system. Each medical problem will be discussed separately with an illustrative case history.

CASE STUDY OF AN APHASIC

It was the fifth day that Annie felt the pain in her head. There seemed to be a pot of boiling syrup just under the lid of her hair. She had tried to ignore it and meet her daily obligations—keeping house and cooking for her husband, cleaning and shopping for her recently widowed sister who was enfeebled by a heart attack, and working part-time as a bookkeeper in the office of a coal company. She was sitting at the desk now, wishing for ice or a cold cloth to press against her head. Surely it was not a tension headache. Although she had become an expert in tension and worry in the two years since her brother-in-law first became ill, his death had brought a certain relief. Without the hospital visits the pace of her daily activity had slowed down.

The constancy and duration of the pain was mystifying. She could not eat or add figures, and she could barely answer the telephone. In the middle of the afternoon, she imagined she was on top of a mountain in a snowstorm. But her calendar said August 3. The strangeness of the delusion jolted her into action. She dialed her doctor and then the shop where her husband worked.

Annie was admitted to the hospital that evening. Over the next three days she submitted to a variety of diagnostic tests while her headache persisted. The neurologist discovered an aneurysm in the left temporal parietal region of her brain. An aneurysm is a dilation or bubbling out of the wall of a blood vessel, in Annie's case of the internal carotid artery. A blood flow study revealed dead tissue in that area of the brain, but the aneurysm had sealed itself off from the main channel without doing further damage.

When the pain subsided Annie noticed weakness in her right arm and hand. Even after months of physical therapy some paralysis remained in the hand and fingers. Writing and typing became awkward, left-handed activities.

Communication was an immediate problem. What little talking she did right after the trauma was gibberish. She tried to telephone her sister but could not be understood. A speech pathologist administered the Boston Diagnostic Examination for Aphasia and found several disturbances. Annie's primary deficit was expressive language: she was unable to retrieve appropriate words or to generate complete sentences. Her articulatory muscles were not impaired, and the first intelligible message she expressed was multisyllabic: "I'm ambulatory."

Patients with damage in the posterior margin of the language area typically show reading and writing deficits. Annie did too. She had visual confusions, and her reading comprehension was barely functional. She had difficulty beyond the undeveloped dexterity of the left hand in writing alphabet letters from dictation, especially the letter "r."

The speech pathologist also administered a hearing screening test and found that sense to be well within normal limits. Annie's ability to understand conversation moved from mild impairment to no impairment within 3 months.

Many psychosocial changes occurred after the trauma. With advancing physical recovery, there was increased mental awareness of the losses. There was a period of emotional lability—laughing and crying jags—and the frustration and embarrassment of being unable to express oneself. After she was released from the hospital, Annie fell into a deep depression. She could not reconcile her changed body image with the demands of life in the kitchen, the bathroom, and the bedroom. Yet she did not remain bitter and secluded. The same sense of family obligation that drove her to tension headaches was reciprocated by her sister and husband. Although she never returned to her job, she managed the family's bookkeeping, housework, and modest social life. She spoke well, with only slight hesitancy as she sought for unfamiliar words. With the ability to drive a car, she became active in volunteer work, including the county stroke club.

EFFECTS OF STROKE .

Strokes or cerebrovascular accidents (CVAs) are the most common cause of brain damage to adults. In fact, doctors often refer to stroke as a "brain attack" and try to get as much special care for those patients as for heart attack patients. While it is the third leading cause of death in the United States, it is the first cause of adult disability.

"Vascular," as a term, refers to blood vessels, arteries, and veins. A stroke is an interference with the blood supply to the brain causing abnormalities of tissue, called lesions. Recovery is rarely, if ever, complete, and loss of function of any amount of brain tissue can leave the individual with defects in thinking, personality, and motor or sensory function.

The American Stroke Association reports that 600,000 new strokes occur every year in the United States, and two thirds of them occur in people age 65 and over. There is a residual population of nearly three million survivors who have neurologic deficits. Despite the accumulation of a large body of knowledge about brain circulation and metabolism, central nervous system function, and arteriosclerosis, nothing has been discovered that will reduce the area of cerebral damage once it has occurred or will promote regeneration of defunct nervous tissue.

Efforts to prevent stroke can be successful. The public education campaign launched against hypertension (high blood pressure) is cited as an important factor in the reduced incidence of stroke. The Federal Drug Administration's approval of tissue plasminogen activator (TPA) also reduced deaths. If given within 3 hours after the onset of a stroke it can dissolve the blood clot. Aspirin therapy has also been credited with preventing blood clots. Because of these innovations the number of stroke deaths nationwide has declined by approximately 5% per year.

There are several types of CVAs. In thrombosis, clotted blood or scar tissue from vessel walls can build up and block off an area of the brain from the flow of nutrition and oxygen that blood carries. The effects of embolism are similar. In embolism, the clogging factor is a bit of blood, fat, air, or bacteria traveling from some other location, rather than building up at the site. Sometimes a blood vessel breaks and bleeds into the brain. This is called intracerebral hemorrhage.

Other, less frequent causes of brain damage in adults are tumors, head injuries (as from war or auto accidents), toxins, and infections or degenerative diseases. The extent and the location of the brain damage determines what neurologic functions will be lost. Patients may show similar symptoms even though the precipitating cause was different.

The brain consists of two fairly similar halves—a right hemisphere and a left hemisphere. They exert contralateral (opposite-sided) control over the activities of the body—both sensory and motor. For instance, visual impulses to the right eye are perceived in the left occipital lobe, an area of the cerebrum known to receive stimuli from the eye. Brain damage in the motor areas of the right hemisphere produces paralysis in the left arm or leg. While children below the age of puberty may be fairly plastic in laterality, adults become more habituated to their dominant hemisphere year by year.

In most people, the left side of the brain is dominant in the control of speech, language, and right hand dexterity. Of the 10%

of the adult population that have right hemisphere or mixed dominance for motor activity, about two-thirds have left hemisphere control for language (Moskovitch, 1976).

Aphasia

Aphasia, or dysphasia (the prefix dys implies less than total loss of
function), is the consequence of left hemisphere damage. It is a
disorder of the capacity to deal with all aspects of symbolic language—verbal, gestural, visual, and graphic. Reading, writing, and
computation deficits are a sign of aphasia, not loss of intelligence.
Twenty-five percent of all stroke patients (about 80,000 individuals)
develop some type of aphasia each year (NIDCD, 1997).

A description of the symptom complex of aphasia can be simplified
by dividing it into two major types, expressive and recessive. Predominantly expressive aphasia is a disturbance in the ability to formulate
and encode ideas symbolically. Patients have trouble remembering
specific words and grammatical forms. Often the message comes out
like a telegram (key words only) delivered by a balking automaton.
Abstract vocabulary with intangible connotations is most likely to be
lost. Automatic phrases, swearing, and slang appear over and over
again, in the wrong places, at the wrong times.

Predominantly receptive aphasia is difficulty in the comprehension of spoken or written language. Patients cannot understand what
the doctors, nurses, or family say about the illness, though they may
gain some information from nonverbal cues. Directions must be
repeated or acted out for them unless they have some residual reading ability. Often receptive aphasia interferes with self-hearing. A
fluent aphasic can be unaware that his/her free-flowing sentences
amount to incomprehensible jargon to the listener. Yet, the hearing
mechanism is physically intact.

Aphasic persons also have trouble with the two functions of memory—retention and recall. Retention is the storing up of what has
been learned, and recall is the use of what has been stored. The
person may lose part of what is stored, as well as losing the ability
to draw particular memories out of storage. The name of the hospital
or of one's partner can be forgotten early in the poststroke period.
Old personal memories return first, and for immigrants that might

mean reversion to the language of childhood. Memory for recent events may take a long time to reappear.

Regaining the ability to communicate is a high priority for people who have had a stroke. They need language to carry on the routine activities of daily life and also to regain their social/emotional lives. New models of health care combine biomedical and social science knowledge to offer patients a reasonable quality of life. So speech-language pathologists have developed a 7-level scale for functional communication. It starts with mere alertness, moves to responding to yes/no questions, then to following simple directions without cues, to understanding limited conversation with familiar people, to initiating conversations in vocational, avocational, and social settings (Frattali, 1998).

Individualized, one-on-one speech-language therapy can be costly in terms of time and resources, so the Aphasia Center of California made a careful study of group treatment (Elman & Bernstein, 1999). Groups were balanced for age, education level, and severity of aphasia. Fifty participants received 5 hours of group work each week for 4 months. All members scored higher on communicative and linguistic measures than the control group. Further, there was no decline in performance in a follow-up study 4 months after treatment had ended.

Behavior changes frequently take place in aphasic patients. Depression and frustration at the inability to communicate may lead to withdrawal. Lethargy, limited attention span, and self-centeredness may replace their former sociability. They may become excessively rigid and adhere to a strict schedule for meals and medicine. Emotional lability (broad mood swings) is to be expected. They cry or laugh very easily, act depressed or elated, and cooperate or balk within short periods of time. Such behavior is not willful but is a consequence of the brain damage. It declines with recovery and rehabilitation.

Agnosia

Another concomitant of stroke or brain tumor is agnosia. This is a problem of not knowing the significance of an incoming sensory stimulus. For instance, victims of aphasia may also suffer auditory agnosia. Their ears hear, but the sounds are not properly perceived in the brain. They hear a ring but do not glance toward the telephone or the door. They hear words and phrases but are deaf to their meaning.

Although agnosia is not a language disorder as such, it is further confused when aphasia exists with it. Family members, and even examiners, tend to rely on what the patient says to indicate the brain's grasp of sensory input. Sometimes patients cannot name an object but can draw it or select it by touch from a group of objects.

Agnosias are named for the specific sensory modality that is affected, such as touch, vision, or hearing. There are many abstruse terms, such as topographagnosia (the inability to read maps), but they can be classified under the three main headings of visual agnosia, auditory agnosia, and tactile agnosia. When a stroke damages only the right hemisphere, the victim may suffer agnosias for spatial relations and form. Posterior left hemisphere damage is associated with auditory agnosia.

Apraxia

Another consequence of brain damage is apraxia. It is a difficulty in the voluntary programming of oral motor movements in the absence of muscle impairment. In oral apraxia, for example, patients may not be able to whistle or lick their lips on request, but they might perform those tasks later on, automatically. After eating, the lips may be licked quite effortlessly and unconsciously.

Articulatory apraxia is the term for disturbance of voluntary speech movements. About half of clients with aphasia also suffer from articulatory apraxia. The most noticeable symptom is the struggle behavior as the apraxic tries to position tongue and lips to form the desired sound. This slows down and breaks the rhythm of speech. The sounds pronounced are likely to be errors and occur in the wrong order (e.g., "flatporms" instead of "platforms").

There is little consistency in the sound errors, as there would be if actual, specific muscles were impaired. Errors tend toward simplification. Long words and words with consonant clusters cause the most trouble, so in diagnostic tests key words like "statistician" and "Methodist Episcopal" are elicited. Repetitions like "statition" would reveal apraxic involvement.

CASE STUDY OF A DYSARTHRIC

Dan did not know he was becoming a statistic for one of the most common neurologic diseases of the aged (two per 100 over age 60). He only knew that his hands shook and he could not seem to straighten up and march down the aisle at church with his former erect posture. And, while passing the collection plate, the fingers of his free hand seemed to be rolling little balls. Hadn't he seen that in an old World War II movie? He remembered Humphrey Bogart as the commander whose nervous hands belied his testimony in The Caine Mutiny Court Martial. Was he having a mental breakdown too?

He got up his courage and made an appointment with the neurologist his family doctor recommended. After a lengthy examination, Dan learned that he was a victim of Parkinson's disease. Annually 50,000 people are diagnosed with the condition and 10% of those are under age 40 (Lieberman, 1998). This degenerative neuromuscular disease was going to slow down and limit his range of movement, bend his proud stance, shuffle his confident stride, and solidify his facial expression. His speech, when he could jerk those muscles into action, would be slower, softer, and less intelligible. But Parkinson's would not disturb his intellect. He was grateful that his ability to think was preserved, and he used it to decide on a course of action.

Although surgery could freeze out the malfunctioning cells of the basal ganglia in his brain, he chose a more conservative treatment—medication. Since his own brain was failing to produce enough dopamine—the chemical substance thought to aid transmission of nerve messages—he would take L-dopa. In fact, there was a new drug that contained the beneficial L-dopa plus inhibitors for some of the unpleasant side effects like nausea. The levodopa/cardidopa combination was marketed as Sinemet or Lodosyn.

For young-onset patients who take L-dopa for 5 years or more and develop wild, involuntary movements, pharmacists have developed less noxious drugs. A well-calibrated drug regimen may give a patient 10 or more good years, but the miracles eventually wear out. So treatment becomes removal of small masses of brain tissue or implanting electrodes wired to a battery-powered stimulator that the patient controls (Cowley, 2000).

In the past decade another path of relief was found. Scores of patients regained use of their bodies after fetal cell implantation.

Surgeons graft fetal dopamine-producing cells into the striatum. Stem cells could be cultivated to do the same function (Cowley, 2000). Personally, Dan felt squeamish about such procedures.

Having spent over 30 years of his life as an industrial salesman Dan had incorporated parts of that stereotype into his own self-image. He believed that the way he dressed, moved, and spoke revealed his prosperity and confidence. His self-image showed pride in himself, his product, and his company. Tall and handsome already, he had adopted a rapid, energetic way of walking and talking. It was just these characteristics that had drawn a much younger woman to marry him after his first wife died. How would he meet her expectations now?

Fortunately, L-dopa treatment was effective, and the gross motor symptoms were reduced. Yet, Dan was shrewd enough to know that prolonged treatment might not be consistently satisfactory. He wanted insurance for the speaking mechanism that made it possible for him to sell, to maintain his sociability, and to reveal his mental astuteness. He faithfully attended a speech therapy group that worked on dysarthria—the collective term for the weakness, paralysis, or incoordination of the speech muscles. The medical causes were diverse—stroke, multiple sclerosis, bulbar palsy, muscular dystrophy, amyotrophic lateral sclerosis (ALS), tumors, even alcohol toxicity—but the therapy was basically the same. The goal was to increase intelligibility by increasing loudness and oral movements and by controlling melody, rate, and syllable stress. With his good motivation and intellectual grasp of the process, Dan became an inspiring model to other group members. Once again, he was selling himself and a process—successfully.

EFFECTS OF MEDICAL CONDITIONS

Dysarthria is a problem in the voluntary muscular control of the speech mechanism. When the central nervous system or the peripheral nervous system is damaged, the body parts used in producing speech are affected. For instance, breathing muscles may be weakened, slowed, or poorly coordinated forcing the speaker to use short, gaspy phrases. The muscles for phonating, articulating, and resonating may be affected in the same way. The result will be unintelligible speech. The degree of unintelligibility will be directly related to the severity of the dysarthria. The presenting problem is poor oral speech, but inner language and thinking may be as sharp as before.

When the dysarthria is caused by central nervous system damage, location of the lesion is a key determinant. The stroke victim who has damage to only one hemisphere will be more intelligible than someone who has bilateral damage in the motor control areas. The explanation lies in the fact that the muscles for speech are innervated by both hemispheres. When neuromotor conditions are still developing, a trained speech pathologist is a key informant to the neurologist who must make a diagnosis. Many an insidious brain tumor first reveals itself in disordered speech. Because speech pathologists have trained hearing and analytical skills, they can deduce from the progressive deterioration in speech where the tumor is growing. Table 4.1 contrasts the symptoms and management of apraxia and dysarthria.

The detective work described above is possible because of the pioneering research of Darley, Aronson, and Brown (1975). They have classified six forms of dysarthria and listed the breathing, phonating, and articulating deviations for each symptom type. The types of dysarthria are flaccid, spastic, ataxic, hypokinetic, hyperkinetic, and mixed. The symptoms for each do not depend on the causative disease itself but on what location in the nervous system the disease strikes. Either an inflammation, a tumor, or a toxic injection to a particular nerve would all result in the same malfunction of the muscles controlled by that nerve. Two types will be described to show the range of dysarthria.

1. Flaccid dysarthria refers to the speech problems caused by lower motor neuron damage. The muscles are flabby, feeble, or paralyzed. The presenting disease may be bulbar palsy, muscular dystrophy, myasthenia gravis, or others, but the effects on speech are similar. The weakened respiratory system decreases loudness and pitch variability and shortens phrases. The weakened laryngeal muscles can cause "breathy" voice quality, double pitches, and vocalized inhalation (part of the sound you hear when someone snores). A weakened soft palate allows nasal emission of air and too much nasal resonance. Weakened

TABLE 4.1   Motor Speech Problems

<table>
<tr><td colspan="4" align="center">Dysarthria</td></tr>
<tr><td>Medical Case
History</td><td>Nature of
Damage</td><td>Symptoms</td><td>Management</td></tr>
<tr>
<td>CVA (stroke)
TIA (transient
stroke)
Head Trauma
(injury)
Brain Tumor
Parkinson's
Disease
Amyotrophic Lat-
eral Sclerosis
(Lou Gehrig's
Disease)</td>
<td>• Injury or de-
generation of
the neurologi-
cal systems
that control
the muscles
needed for
oral speech
• Neuromotor
functioning of
other body
parts can be
impaired
• Specific symp-
toms depend
on location of
damage
• Co-occurs
with some
types of
aphasia</td>
<td>• Weakness,
slowness, in-
coordination of
muscles used
for speech,
swallowing,
and eating
• Slurred
articulations
• Inconsistent
misarticulation
• Unusual into-
nation, speech
rate, and
stress patterns
• Tremor and ex-
plosive
movements
• Vocal quality
can be harsh,
hoarse, or
nasal</td>
<td>• Train patient
to be more in-
telligible by
slowing
speed, short-
ening mes-
sages, and
increasing ar-
ticulation effort
• Use compen-
satory equip-
ment, such as
electronic de-
vices or com-
munication
boards
• Encourage pa-
tient to write
messages</td>
</tr>
</table>

(continued)

tongue, lips, and jaw slow down the rate of movement and impair the accuracy of sound production. The use of the oral structures for eating—chewing and swallowing—is negatively affected, too.

2. Ataxic dysarthria refers to the speech problems caused by damage to the cerebellum, the part of the brain that regulates force, speed, timing, range, and direction of movement. The presenting condition may be a tumor, multiple sclerosis, encephalitis, cerebrovascular accident, or others. The breathing and phonatory symptoms are reduced range of pitch and loudness and intermittent "bursts" of vocal effort. Articulation is

TABLE 4.1 *(continued)*

		Apraxia	
Medical Case History	Nature of Damage	Symptoms	Management
CVA Head Trauma Brain Tumor	• Damage close to Broca's area of frontal lobe • Only motoric programming for speech is affected • Vegetative functions and unconscious speech movements are not affected • Co-occurs with some types of aphasia	• Inconsistent additions and substitutions of sounds when producing words • Hesitations, restarts, and repetitions of words and sounds • Automatic messages (greeting) better than thoughtful speech	• Encourage patient to write • Use compensatory equipment, such as electronic devices or communication boards

inaccurate and irregular; sounds and pauses are prolonged erratically. The speech symptoms give the general impression that the speaker is drunk from alcohol.

Medical science has added years to the life of our geriatric population, even to those who suffer degenerative neurological diseases. There are no comprehensive incidence figures for the various types of dysarthria, but the category as a whole will increase as brain diseases become more manageable. Patients who survive will need help in overcoming the social and communicative problems that follow the disease.

Dysarthria can be treated in a variety of ways. Whether the presenting disease is progressive or static, the physician may use surgery or drug therapy to promote adjustment. Physical therapy may improve the function of various muscles. Mechanical devices such as a prosthetic palate to control hypernasality may be fitted to support weakened muscles.

Biofeedback machines can help victims monitor their own body processes. By watching a visual display of the electrical activity in contracting muscles, the dysarthric can vary and control the amount of relaxation and tension.

For severe dysarthrics whose arm and hand muscles are unaffected, portable computers can be operated by mouse, trackball, or touch screen. Outfitted with language application software, users can put out written messages or synthesized speech (Romich, 2000). Severely impaired patients can still access E-mail, webpages, word processing, and other text applications by infrared headpointers or switches. The latter can be operated at various levels of force. Wobble switches are activated by gross movements; pneumatic switches respond to a user puffing air out, or sipping air in; very small switches can be operated by controlled movement of tongue, nose, or chin. Other nonverbal devices range from communication boards with pictures, words, or alphabet letters to portable electronic voice synthesizers.

Direct treatment for oral speech production involves working on respiration, phonation, resonation, and articulation to the extent each process is affected. To compensate for neurological damage, clients may have to exaggerate articulatory movements, emphasize all syllables, and slow down overall rate of speaking.

Concentration improves speech production, but sustained effort is fatiguing. Patients should not be expected to overtax themselves to communicate. Reasonable expectations are derived from data on general health and energy level.

CASE STUDY OF A LARYNGECTOMEE

Lance looked like a tough traffic cop who was getting a little portly with the passing years. His muscular chest and shoulders still dominated his body frame, which was just at average height. He had never worked outside, but in an iron foundry, and the traffic he directed was the job operations of the workers at the foundry. No steelworkers are cream puffs, so Lance used to shout, push, and shove to get things done.

All during that winter of unusually heavy snows, Lance suffered from colds, coughs, and hoarseness. He felt pain not only in his throat but also in his ears. And exertion made him short of breath. His wife worried, and Lance was worried, too. He was on the verge of cutting down on that pack-a-day of cigarettes. Instead, he decided to go to his doctor. This general physician diagnosed the condition as chronic laryngitis, but wisely referred Lance to an ear, nose, and throat (ENT) specialist.

In the laryogoscopic exam, the ENT specialist found a large tumor on the left cord. The doctor removed a section of it to test for malignancy. The cells proved to be cancerous. If the tumor had been smaller, perhaps it could have been treated with X-rays or conservation surgery—a partial removal of the voice mechanism. As it was, Lance was immediately scheduled for a total laryngectomy. The entire larynx from the base of the tongue to the windpipe would have to be removed.

In preoperative counseling, Lance was assured that laryngeal cancer was the most curable of all cancers. It attacks seven men for every woman and totals 13,000 cases a year in the United States. Intervention with radiation, chemotherapy, and/or surgery saves 9500 lives annually. Lance's prognosis was better than for other 62 year olds (the average age for surgical removal of larynx), because he had no hearing loss or other debilities. His proud, gutsy personality and the active roles he played at home and on the job were indicators of early rehabilitation.

In a total laryngectomy, the trachea is drawn forward and sutured to an opening at the base of the neck. This is called the stoma. Since the airflow no longer goes through the mouth and nose, and the vocal cords that would have been vibrated are missing, there is no hope of regaining normal speech.

At first, Lance was more concerned with survival than speech. He felt constant anxiety about choking. Mucus and other secretions accumulated at the stoma, and he was afraid that he might block the hole by accident when he was sleeping.

After the food tube was removed, Lance looked forward to eating a choice steak, but it did not taste the same. As a moderate drinker, he looked forward to a cold beer, but now that did not taste or smell so good. While his own olfactory sense had declined, his wife's was as sharp as ever. She noticed mouth odor, which the nurse eliminated by showing Lance how to brush his tongue and palate as well as his teeth. In this period, Lance lost over 50 pounds of the extra weight he had accumulated over the years.

As Lance's physical health improved, he felt more and more need to communicate. His doctor agreed with him that further surgery, whether to reconstruct a larynx or to implant an electronic device, was not necessary. So Lance tried an artificial, handheld, electro-larynx. He shaped words over the generated buzz, and some of the hospital staff understood him, but his wife objected to the robot sound. She appeared to be a tough-spirited, but loving person, al-though new fears overwhelmed her. She did not want to face her husband's early retirement nor drastic changes in their social life. To calm herself, she crocheted gorgets (the small bibs worn over the stoma to warm and filter the incoming air) and made plans for Lance's rehabilitation.

About 3 weeks after surgery, Lance was introduced to the speech pathologist who demonstrated esophageal speech. It involves swal-lowing air and regurgitating it. The air bubble vibrates the sphincter muscles at the top of the food pipe, thus producing a brief tone. Lance accepted the explanations in a matter-of-fact way, but just could not begin. When the clinician encouraged him to visualize his last bottle of beer, he closed his eyes and emitted a gurgled "good."

Although Lance was well motivated, he did not have much pa-tience. He learned about a voice prosthesis from a support group on the Internet. When the ENT examined him for suitability, a second surgery was performed. Not only did he prefer the new voice, but Lance also found that the device was easy to install, clean, and maintain. He could wear the same prosthesis 24 hours a day, 7 days a week for 3–4 months with no problems.

EFFECTS OF SURGERY

The most severe vocal problem that can happen to an older person is cancer of the larynx. If it is detected in the early stages, it can be treated with chemotherapy, radiation, or surgery limited to the exact site (perhaps one vocal cord) (Weinstein, 1999). Extensive malignan-cies require removal of the whole larynx and creation of a permanent tracheostoma (hole in the front of the neck) for breathing. The National Cancer Institute (2000) reports that there are 50,000 laryngectomees in the United States and the majority of them have returned to society as useful citizens.

Persistent hoarseness is one of the commonest symptoms of a developing pathology. Other signs are pain in the throat or ear, frequent throat clearing, and shortness of breath. Certain habits of daily living contribute to the chance of cancer. They are heavy smoking and loud and excessive talking in environments where the air is contaminated with smoke and particulate matter.

Although the greatest problem postoperatively is the lack of voice, patients have to make an immediate adaptation to their new breathing system. They must learn how to keep the stoma open and clean. The use of kerchiefs, crocheted bibs, or turtleneck sweaters is not merely a cosmetic device to avoid curious stares. Those coverings filter out dust particles and warm the air before it enters the trachea. Eating habits may have to change in the direction of softer food if swallowing is difficult. The senses of smell and taste are less acute, since mouth and nose are no longer a part of the breathing system. Bad breath can occur, too, and is reduced by brushing tongue and palate as well as teeth on a routine basis. Bathing and showering (with a shield to keep water out of the stoma) are daily rituals and swimming is impossible.

An artificial larynx is one way to regain speech. There are pneumatic and electronic types. The first carries air from the lungs to the mouth through a tube. The second is a battery-powered, hand-held device whose vibrating diaphragm is pressed against the soft tissues of the neck. A cosmetic variation of the electronic larynx is a pipe with the battery mounted neatly beneath the bowl. Visible or not, many laryngectomees object to the battery-run device, because its operating tone makes them sound like robots.

Another method is esophageal speech. This involves taking air into the upper part of the food pipe and adapting those normal sphincter muscles to vibrate like vocal cords. Of course, without the former large air supply and supporting laryngeal structures, this tone does not sound normal. It is soft, low-pitched, and monotonic. It sounds like a burp. But that tone can be extended, resonated, and shaped by the articulators into intelligible speech. Esophageal speech requires no batteries and both hands are free for other activities.

The disadvantages of esophageal speech may be particularly inhib-iting for the elderly. First, the process of learning is difficult and time-consuming. Second, the tone produced is not loud, and if the laryngectomee has hearing loss, self-monitoring is difficult. Devel-oping intelligibility of the esophageal tone requires sharp hearing. Furthermore, if the spouse or other listeners have hearing loss, the laryngectomee will not be understood very well.

In the 1980s, a handy shortcut to generating that "burp" was devised. It begins with a secondary surgery. The doctor makes a small hole from the rear of the stoma to the esophagus, a tracheo-esophageal puncture (TEP). After healing, a small plastic prosthetic device is inserted into a puncture from the trachea to the esophagus. By closing the stoma with the thumb or a special valve, air flowing out of the lungs is shunted over into the food pipe where esophageal muscles produce phonation. That sound is shaped into words in the normal manner. This Blom-Singer prosthesis has a one-way valve to prevent swallowed food and liquid from entering the air passageway.

In Britain surgeons frequently perform the TEP during the origi-nal laryngectomy and insert the prosthesis (Provox 2) at that time (Davidson, 1998). To insure success patients must have anatomic suitability, manual dexterity, visual acuity, good stoma hygiene, and motivation. With the prosthesis in place, 91% of the patients develop good-quality, effortless speech.

A small percentage of laryngectomees seem unable to speak at all. Rather than suffering in silence, they can adapt to using nonverbal means, such as writing, communication boards, or voice synthesizers. Keeping contact with others is essential to morale. The longer the postoperative life expectancy, the greater the need for establishing some means of communication to promote self-expression, self-care, and social interaction.

FAMILY'S REACTION

The family, whether it is a partner, surviving siblings, or grown children, can be deeply affected by an older person's illness. They are concerned about the health problem, the functional level of recovery, the length of hospitalization, and the cost of extended care. The socioeconomic concerns are no less worthy than personal ones, as the latter can be prompted by guilt or fear for one's own well-being.

Crises have been said to draw a family closer together. That is most often the case. Family members visit and stay close during the crucial period of hospitalization, even though they may not be competent to help. Quietly and anxiously, they wait for a patient to regain conscious memory or recognition. In lucid moments, the patient is heartened by their presence.

During convalescence, reliable family members can carry out specific treatments. As their self-control and knowledge of the illness increases, their assistance and observations become more and more valuable. Constructive activities relieve the frustration, anger, or grief the crisis precipitated. During the period of rehabilitation, the patient suffers such emotional upset that the only anchor is family. The stability, patience, and determined optimism displayed by a loved one can have phenomenal healing power.

The American Heart Association (2000) recommends that families give enough help so the aphasic person does not become frustrated, but not so much that he/she becomes overly dependent. Further, the person should be treated as a mature and responsible adult and share in life decisions. The family can help by offering stimulating and understanding companionship. If patients are continually left by themselves, their language progress slows down, they withdraw, and they grow more depressed and anxious. Stimulation arouses the patient to make efforts toward rehabilitation.

Yet caregivers need to vent their own negative emotions. They can talk with friends, health care professionals, counseling psychologists, or clergy. The American Stroke Association maintains a Warmline at 1-800-553-6321 to meet this need.

While the laryngectomee must conquer the grief of losing a body part and any aversion to the sound of esophageal speech, the dysarthric must face the prospect of progressive disability. Many of the diseases associated with dysarthria are incurable, and remission of symptoms through medication or therapy is the most that can be expected. In addition to the depression and anxiety suffered by all elderly ill people, the victim of Parkinson's disease has a fear of falling due to awkwardness. Body image is changed due to slowness and unreliability of the muscles. Family members have to alter their environment (remove door sills and fragile lamps) and use great patience and tact to stimulate independence. Parkinsonism is best held at bay by keeping the muscles in action by doing ordinary chores, no matter how long it takes.

Although most families rally to a crisis, some are rejecting. Those families are so caught up in their own needs and problems that they refuse to accept the patient or the illness. Grown children may be at a stage in their own lives that exacerbates natural fears of death or disability. The male in mid-life crisis may be too concerned for his own health and virility to acknowledge the vulnerability of his parents. The female may already be overburdened with caregiving roles as a mother, a grandmother, or other guardian. Accepting the dependence of the elderly is almost more devastating than accepting their mortality. It entails more responsibility and serves as a constant reminder that the cocoon of childhood and the dreams of youth are gone forever. When the family does not take up burdens, the chances of later regret and guilt increase.

ANXIETY AND DEPRESSION

The elderly ill are at great risk for mental health problems. They are prone to anxiety and depression and the resultant agitation makes other people uncomfortable. Because there is medication available to treat these problems they may be over-diagnosed (Bell, 1999). Since some drugs are addictive and cause serious side effects the symptoms should have lasted 6 months and caused significant interference with everyday life before drugs are prescribed.

Anxiety and depression are both liaisons of living. They can coexist in the same person at normal or clinical levels. For instance, a family caregiver to both parents had a double burden of stress. Her father had vascular dementia brought on by TIA's (transient ischemic attacks). In his lucid periods he expressed the bitter and depressing thoughts that plagued him. Her mother had late-onset Alzheimer's Disease and seemed to be living in her own world (a world that existed when she was age 13). But she wore a small frown of anxiety as she wandered aimlessly from project to project, undertaking household chores without rhyme or reason, and quickly forgetting them.

Despite genetic predictions, the daughter claimed to be unconcerned about her own future: "In the mornings I lean toward my mother's behavior—high energy and only middling direction, but in the afternoons I resemble my father—morose and depleted. I can go either way and I'm glad I don't have to make the decision."

The most common emotional problem is depression. It reaches clinical significance in 12–16% of the medically ill and persons in long-term care (Blazer, 1997). It is a corollary to fear of death and disability and to the increasing losses of highly valued people, objects, and relationships. Widows discover that their husbands were the habit of a lifetime. They feel a constant, vague unease. The spouse may be forgotten as a person, but not forgotten as a presence. Depressive symptoms are fully delineated in the Diagnostic and Statistical Manual of Mental Disorders, 4th edition (DSM-IV; American Psychiatric Association, 1994). Some are measurable and some are self-reported. They include poor eating and sleeping patterns, despair, lethargy, disinterest, and psychosomatic complaints. Depressed persons feel helpless, hopeless, unwanted, and unloved. When depression is not alleviated, it can lead to suicide. It is a well-known fact that the suicide rate in the United States is highest for the over-65 age group. Older white males are especially prone to solve their physical and emotional problems in this way.

Anxiety is a painful, nonspecific uneasiness of mind over an impending or anticipated unpleasantness. At low levels, it can spur one to take constructive remedial action; at high levels it can cripple any effective functioning. In terms of communication, the anxious patient can be abrupt or distant, or nervously voluble. Some of the physical signs of anxiety are sweaty palms, pinpoint pupils, frequent urination, digestive disturbances, trembling, muscular tension, and elevated pulse, respiration, and blood pressure.

Older adults tend to attribute the signs of anxiety to physical illness and many self-diagnosed "heart attacks" are actually panic attacks. Imagining the worst (catastrophizing) is a common symptom of generalized anxiety disorder (GAD). Fearing hospitalization or institutionalization, the oldsters avoid treatment (Stanley & Averill, 1999).

Fortunately, both anxiety and depression can be alleviated through medication. Anti-anxiety drugs like Valium, a benzodiasepine, have the risk of addiction, so anxious persons may be given an antidepressant. Selective serotonin-reuptake inhibitors (SSRIs) are proving to be effective and have minor side effects (MDConsult, 2000). Table 4.2 summarizes the observable contrasts between anxious persons and depressed persons.

The major problem with drug treatment for emotional problems is noncompliance. Once patients feel better they stop taking pills. Or they object to side effects that make the body feel worse, even though the mood is improved. Some antidepressants take 2–4 weeks before they are fully effective and then are retained in the body for weeks after the last pill is taken. The elimination half-life of benzodiazepines is 3 times longer in old persons compared to younger persons (Blazer, 1997). Newer, short-acting drugs like busipirones are less likely to have negative side effects. Patients object to confusion, morning "hangover," slurred speech, and problems with balance and coordination. Consequently, the general rule for elderly clients is to prescribe the lowest effective dose and to monitor it carefully.

Treating the causes of affective disorders helps reduce symptoms and drug use. Group or individual psychotherapy, desensitization, relaxation, and modeling are popular approaches. Cognitive-behav-

TABLE 4.2 Symptoms Typical of Anxious and Depressed Persons

Observable Traits	Anxious Person	Depressed Person
Communication style	Verbalizes emotions Elaborates problems	Avoids conversation Offers little information
Attitude toward life	Participates impulsively	Acts resigned
Time orientation	Anticipates the future	Reverts to the past
Activity patterns	Active early in the day	Active late in the day
Eating habits	Enjoys meals for socializing May eat compulsively	Loss of weight and appetite May eat compulsively
Gastrointestinal response	Diarrhea	Constipation
Pulse, respiration, and blood pressure	Raised vital signs	Lowered vital signs
Medication	Takes "downers," tranquilizers, Buspar	Takes "uppers," selective serotonin uptake inhibitors (SSRIs), Prozac

ioral therapy (CBT) can become effective in 12–20 weeks. It breaks up the entrenched negative thoughts (ruminations) by sharpening the person's self-observation. Clients "see" the realities of problem situations and respond with new actions based on reasonable expectations. People of all ages ask for a "reality check" when events seem overwhelming. So CBT works well as part of overall treatment.

THERAPEUTIC RELATIONSHIP

The goals of therapeutic relationships are to build trust, to relieve anxiety, and to increase understanding. When a professional communicates with the elderly ill those goals are in mind even though the interchange appears to be mere social conversation.

Building trust with an ill person requires kindness and faithfulness. It does not necessarily require a lot of time as long as the professional sets and keeps definite times for a visit. Reliability counts. Attention and supportive listening can help the depressed take a more realistic look at themselves. Responses must not belittle the problems and feelings they confide to you. Glib attempts to allay worries and cajole them into a lighter mood seem only to discount the validity of their emotions. If they feel cared about as well as cared for, if they feel spoken with as well as spoken to, and if they feel respected for their basic personality, residual strengths, and past achievements, they will respond cooperatively.

Supportive communication can help relieve free-floating anxiety by reaffirming the value of each person as a human being. The patient needs to know that the anxious behavior (verbal and nonverbal) is understandable and acceptable. Whenever possible, giving the dreaded situation a specific name objectifies it and makes it less bewildering. One of the oldest religious traditions of the Anglo-Saxon heritage is "unmasking" at midnight the ghouls and ghosties of All Hallow's Eve. When a feared object, illness, or procedure is named and seen to be real, its familiar qualities can be coped with realistically.

Anxiety involves fear of the unknown, the new, and the future. The French philosopher, Montaigne, averred that anticipation is the magnifying glass of the emotions. Consequently, information about the unknown and preparation for the future are sensible antidotes to anxiety. Some oldsters or their caregivers will go to the library or access the Internet from a home computer. Health sites abound and supply easy to read information. Others seek personal testimony. For example, a visit from a member of the IAL (a support organization for laryngectomees) can inform the preoperative cancer victim about the laryngectomy itself and the success of rehabilitation procedures.

Some hospitals use closed-circuit television to relay appropriate medical information to patients undergoing conventional procedures. They maintain a library of tapes on topics such as baby care, hysterectomy, and tonsils, as well as the medical conditions of the elderly.

While impersonal, one-way videotapes are a convenient way to convey information, they cannot replace the third goal of the therapeutic relationship—increasing understanding. That requires two-way communication. If knowledge is power, then giving knowledge gives the patient power to conquer fear (anxiety) and helplessness (depression).

The ideal health communicator recognizes the patient's right to know but is sensitive to the patient's ability to receive. Timing is a crucial factor. There are high stress periods in an illness when negative emotions dominate reason. Information should be conveyed during relaxed times. It needs to be repeated—for everyone not just "forgetful" oldsters—during a time when there is less static from stress.

Language is another key factor. Medical terms are unfamiliar, latinized, long, and difficult to read, spell, and pronounce. A nonspecialist explanation must be accurate, but jargon-free. Even native speakers of English do not use "book" words for certain body parts, but they understand direct Anglo-Saxon definitions and accept them as authoritative.

Authority of the source of information may affect its reception but does not guarantee compliance. While patients listen to the physician with proper awe, they like to check the facts and interpretation with other care providers with whom they have a personal relationship. The person who has earned their trust and relieved their anxieties is the person whose recommendations they will remember and implement. Because the therapeutic relationship is a whole—a circle of giving and taking—it is more powerful than cold authority. It can give the elderly ill person not only the understanding but also the motivation to recuperate and rehabilitate.

EXERCISES

Worrying Survey

Please fill out this questionnaire for yourself, and then complete the questionnaire a second time with an elderly person acting as the respondent.

1. I know I'm worried when (circle all items that apply):
   a. I can't sleep
   b. Food doesn't interest me
   c. My mind hangs onto the problem
   d. I feel frightened
   e. I don't feel like talking
   f. Other people get on my nerves
   g. Nothing makes me laugh or smile

2. Which bodily reactions do you feel when you are worried?
   a. Headache
   b. "Knot in stomach"
   c. Teary eyes
   d. Rapid breathing
   e. Shaky hands
   f. Slumped posture
   g. Eye squinting
   h. Increased heart rate

3. The things I worry about most are:
   a. Money
   b. My health
   c. The future
   d. My job
   e. My lack of achievements
   f. Health of a loved one
   g. My family's crisis

   h. My current achievement
   i. World crisis

4. When I get in a "worrying mood" it spreads to other parts of my life:
   a. Often
   b. Sometimes
   c. Hardly ever

5. All in all, how much worry do you have in your life today?
   a. Some, but not very much
   b. Almost none
   c. A good deal

6. How would you rate the amount of worrying you do?
   a. More than other people
   b. About the same as other people
   c. Less than other people

7. What do you do when you are worried?
   a. Wait for it to go away
   b. Fight back
   c. Tell someone my problem
   d. Blot it out with alcohol, TV, travel, etc.

8. I can fight off worries when (circle only three items):
   a. I prepare for problems
   b. I have power to control the situation
   c. I analyze their cause
   d. I understand my limits
   e. Someone helps me
   f. Time passes and removes the problem

REFERENCES

American Heart Association (2000). *Caring for someone with aphasia.* Dallas, TX: Author.
American Psychiatric Association (1994). Diagnostic and statistical manual of mental disorders (4th ed., p. 327). Washington, DC: Author.

American Speech-Language & Hearing Association (1999). *Communication facts.* Rockville, MD: Author.

American Stroke Association (1998). *Stroke is a medical emergency.* Dallas, TX: Author.

Bell, I. (1999). A guide to current psychopharmological treatments for affective disorders in older adults: anxiety, agitation, and depression. In M. Duffy (Ed.)., *Handbook of counseling and psychotherapy with older adults* (pp. 562–577). New York: John Wiley & Sons.

Blazer, D. (1997). *Emotional problems in later life.* New York: Springer.

Cowley, G. (2000, May 22). The new war on Parkinson's. *Newsweek,* pp. 50–58.

Darley, F. L., Aronson, A., & Brown, J. R. (1975). *Motor speech disorders.* Philadelphia: W. B. Saunders.

Davidson, P. (1998). Voice restoration protheses: The options. *Nursing Times, 94,* 56–58.

Elman, R., & Bernstein, E. (1999). The efficacy of group communication treatment in adults with chronic aphasia. *Journal of Speech, Language, and Hearing Research, 42*(2), 411–419.

Frattali, C. (1998). Assessing functional outcomes: an overview. *Seminars in Speech and Language, 19*(3), 209–221.

Lieberman, A. (1998). New developments in medical research: NIH and Patient Groups. Hearing. Washington, DC: GPO.

MDConsult (2000, March). *Anxiety disorders: Patient education handout.* [On-line]. Available at http://www.mdconsult.com.

Moskovich, M. (1976). On the representation of language in the right hemisphere of right-handed people. *Brain & Language, 3,* 47–71.

National Institute on Deafness and Other Communication Disorders (1997, August). *Facts Sheet: Aphasia* (NIH Pub No. 97-4257). Bethesda, MD: Author.

National Cancer Institute (2000). *Cancer of the larynx.* (NIH Pub No. 95-1568). Bethesda, MD: Author.

Romich, B. (2000). *Using a communication device: Different methods yield different results.* Wooster, OH: Prentke Romich.

Stanley, M. A., & Averill, P. M. (1999). Strategies for treating generalized anxiety in the elderly. In M. Duffy (Ed.), *Handbook of counseling and psychotherapy with older adults* (pp. 562–577). New York: John Wiley & Sons.

Weinstein, G. S. (1999). *Organ preservation surgery for laryngeal cancer.* San Diego, CA: Singular Publishing Group.

5

Exchanging Messages Despite Barriers

Since the civil rights movement of the 1960s and 1970s, there has been an organized reaction against callous and cursory care of the elderly. Because powerlessness has a negative effect on health, many nursing facilities now follow a Patients' Bill of Rights, and independent oldsters stand up for their rights as consumers of retirement and rehabilitation services.

Although the right to talk may be the beginning of freedom, it is worthless to talk if nobody will listen. Some elderly people love to talk, because they feel secure when they can hear their own voices. Others are so desperate to establish a two-way interpersonal relation that they overdo and flood the listener with verbiage. Yet they need a good listener who takes a vigorous human interest in what is being told.

MODIFYING YOUR RECEPTION

Listening is a complex combination of hearing and understanding. It depends on, but is not limited to, the physical ability to hear. It also involves the willingness to pay attention and to open mental channels to the speaker's message. In getting set to be a good listener, there are several specific things you can do, physically and attitudinally.

First, you need to arrange your environment. Either remove sources of noise and distraction or remove yourself from their vicinity. For instance, in a recreation room you might ask to make the television softer or you might move into another room. Aphasic persons, among others, communicate best in an environment free of distractions.

Here a few points about respect for people in wheelchairs must be made. First, do not assume that using a wheelchair is a tragedy. Whether permanent or temporary, use is a convenience to allow mobility and conserve energy. The user becomes accustomed to the vehicle and feels uncomfortable if other people lean or hang on the chair. It is a violation of personal space. Furthermore, for an interaction of any length, you should consider sitting down or kneeling to get yourself on the same eye level as the wheelchair user.

Second, you need to adopt the physical posture of attention. Since listening is not merely hearing but involves increased mental activity, it takes energy. It is characterized by faster heart action, quicker circulation of the blood, and a small rise in body temperature. Your body works to process various sensory stimuli from a designated source and to blot out competing distractions.

Hence, some music lovers close their eyes to avoid distracting visual input. Receivers of oral communication, contrarily, have to maintain eye contact with the speaker to enhance listening. Maintaining an alert, upright posture will help you focus your eyes, your ears, and your mind.

Third, you have to prepare yourself attitudinally. Take a vigorous, human interest in what is being said. Self-interest often controls memory: we forget the morning newscast about foreign affairs we cannot control but remember the weather forecast that suggests how many sweaters we need to wear. Find some reason, however tenuous, for listening.

Listening with Brain

Hearing the speaker out is not merely a matter of courtesy. It is an essential step in good listening. The listener who makes snap judgments is usually biased and undisciplined. In the thinking person's world, there are few shortcuts, easy answers, or instant solutions.

If you can circumvent your own psychological blocks and patiently think through the message, you will be able to make better judgments.

While you listen for feelings you are listening, also, for facts. You grasp the general content of the message and the supporting ideas. It is impossible, and unnecessary, to remember every single detail. In your mind, if not out loud, you react, question, and participate.

It is a well-known fact that the rate of speaking is far below the rate of auditory comprehension. People speak at 140 to 180 words per minute, but they think at 300 to 700 words per minute. This rate differential is in your favor. You can understand the speaker and still have four-fifths of your time left for thinking.

The brain reminds you of the speech problems of disabled persons and helps you capitalize on the cues they do give. When apraxic/aphasic clients cannot speak the message, give them paper and pencil to write or draw the idea. Approach them through whatever senses seem relatively unimpaired. Use your brains to compensate for damage to their brains.

Listening with Eyes

People whose listening is impaired by an actual hearing loss learn to compensate by using many cues. Not only do they watch the speaker's lips, but also his/her facial expression, eyes, brow lines, gestures, and posture. From this they flesh out the speaker's full message—intention, conviction, and attitude toward the subject and toward listeners. Listeners with normal hearing also interpret a speaker's nonverbal cues and gain the same knowledge.

Watching for body language helps to close the communication gap. Some gestures yield only general information, but the person who can no longer speak will develop them to send specific messages. In some institutions, formal sign languages (like those used by the Native American or the deaf) are being taught to nonverbal patients. Barring such training, you still learn much by observing a person's gestures with sensitivity and imagination.

Large body movements and posture give you clues about the location and extent of brain damage. They signal probable communication deficits. So do small movements, such as eye blinks and facial tics. Before your ear becomes tuned to a laryngectomee's voice, you may understand him/her by watching the lips.

The nonverbal patient whose language is intact may choose to write a message. The apraxic, the unintelligible dysarthric, and the laryngectomized person who has not yet learned esophageal speech use paper and pencil. Other supplements they can use are a magic slate, a blackboard with magnetized alphabet letters, and a communication board. The latter is a thick sheet of plastic or cardboard with key words and pictures to which the disabled person points. One dexterous stroke victim had magnets put on the small wooden letters that come with the Scrabble game and arranged them on a large cookie pan to spell out messages.

Listening with Ears

The ability to hear is basic to the ability to listen. Even when we hear normally, we seek a quiet, conducive environment that suits the kind of communication transaction we want to have. But when one of the partners has a hearing loss, we need to check the environment for good lighting, too. If he/she can see your lips, facial expression and gestures, the hard-of-hearing person will understand you more readily.

Considering the high incidence of hearing loss in the elderly population, it might be wise to check out the spouse and friends of the laryngectomee. Without vocal cords and the usual supply of air, alaryngeal speech is quite soft, so hard-of-hearing companions are at a disadvantage. In the early stages of rehabilitation, the voice may be no louder than a whisper, and, later, there are definite limits to attainable loudness. Standing as close as 3 to 6 feet and watching the lips will help.

You will notice two other differences when listening to the laryngectomized individual. Phrases are short, because there is no longer any access to the air supply in the lungs. Tone of voice is low-pitched, mechanical, and unmelodic, because other tissues have been adapted to the function of vocal cords.

When dealing with the dysarthric, your ears must be very sharp. Reduced muscular ability makes the speech garbled, indistinct, and dragged out. Listen for a pattern of sound distortions and substitutions. Consistent errors can make a new code. Sometimes, if the patient shortens and repeats the message it becomes more clear. As time goes on, your ear adapts and finds the slow-motion core of intelligibility.

Unfortunately, with the apraxic/aphasic there may be no consistency or core of intelligibility. In contrast, there may be a flow of recognizable but inappropriate words. Your ear receives this but does not accept it at face value. Whether it is fluent jargon or an effortful single word, it may not represent what the aphasic intends to say. During rehabilitation there may be a stage where disconnected words become meaningful. The brain seems to be sending a telegram by using only key words. Your knowledge of the situation and message context will supplement your ears in receiving such messages. Further remedial work may lead to normal sentence usage and more sophisticated language.

Homilies like "actions speak louder than words" or "the truth is in the tone of voice" attest to the fact that words alone do not convey a full message. A careful listener hears and interprets all the nuances of vocal tone and melody pattern. Your friends can tell what kind of day you have had by the sound of your "hello." The sound can lilt or droop. Unfortunately, people who live in institutions tend to develop flat voices. It may indicate a dull, uninteresting life, but more clues would be needed before such a judgment could be made. Certain medications, especially in heavy doses, can affect the quality of vocal tone, too.

Listening with Heart

One of the reasons for listening is to understand the feelings of others. That requires us to listen emphatically—with "heart."

For the ill, it is especially important to maintain a relaxed and friendly manner. Patients who seem nonverbal may be actually asserting themselves: refusing to display their disabilities to someone perceived as cold and brusque. Dysarthrics need your patience because they cannot form the sounds that go into a ready answer. Aphasics need it because they cannot express the words of an answer. Aphasics also experience poorer language comprehension when they feel rushed and embarrassed.

Listening with heart means erasing negative reactions, shock, or condescension. Above all, it is listening acceptingly. Sometimes, hearing emotion-laden words leads to gut reactions. These must be controlled until the full story is heard. A stream of jargon from an aphasic or a resounding belch from a laryngectomee should raise no eyebrows, stir no comment.

See Table 5.1 for ways of listening to elderly persons with speech and/or language disabilities.

MODIFYING YOUR VOCAL PRODUCTION

If only one suggestion could be made for improving your message sending capability, it would be this: slow down. The victims of stroke or hearing loss have difficulty following rapid speech. Other oldsters who feel "slowed down" by the process of aging seem to listen more slowly, too. Most people are quite capable of speaking distinctly when they allow time for the myriad muscle movements involved in speech, so avoiding a rapid rate usually increases your intelligibility.

Not only can you moderate your overall rate of speaking, but you can gain more understanding from listeners by pausing to see if you are understood so far. Listeners need a chance to think and feel the impact of your message. Timely pauses give them that chance.

TABLE 5.1   Summary Chart for Listening to the Elderly Person with Speech/ Language Disabilities: How to Modify Your Listening

For the dysarthric:
  Expect poor articulation, so read gestures and nonverbal cues.
  Listen for the slow motion core of intelligibility.

For the laryngectomee:
  Expect a low-pitched monotone.
  Listen for shortened phrases without melody.
  Listen with your eyes, i.e., lip-read cues.

For the aphasic:
  Listen slowly, i.e., give time for person to grope for words and ideas.
  Listen acceptingly, without negative reactions.
  Expect telegraphic messages from the expressive aphasic.

Since an estimated 39% of older citizens have hearing problems, increasing your loudness is another good technique. Shouting, however, is not helpful, because it tends to raise vocal pitch. The hearing loss of old age typically damages response to high pitch more than response to low pitch. For instance, the hearing impaired person may report difficulty hearing the high-pitched voices of children and some women.

Shouting in someone's ear is a definite mistake. It may violate the sense of personal space and privacy, and it frazzles nerves. One thing it will not do is promote communication. As hearing recedes, a person depends more and more on the sense of sight. Automatically, lip reading begins. He/she tends to read body movements, gestures, and facial expressions as well, so there needs to be good lighting on the speaker's face. Shouting in someone's ear takes you out of the line of vision.

Lip reading will never be a complete solution to hearing loss, because only about a third of the sounds of English are readily visible. An r or g or h is formed too far back in the mouth to be seen. Sounds like b and m are visible, but confusing. Words like "Bobby" and "mopping" look the same on the lips but come from widely different contexts. You can facilitate all possible lip reading if you speak distinctly, but without exaggeration. Avoid chewing, eating, clenching a pipe stem, or covering your mouth with your hands.

A relaxed speaking rate and clear diction will help stroke victims too. The aphasic person needs time to unravel the message, and the apraxic benefits from seeing how the sounds are formed. If the stroke patient has a concomitant hearing loss, your increased loudness aids reception. Although it is preferable to get the listener's attention by motion or a light touch, loudness is a proven way to get and focus attention.

Repeating vs. Rephrasing

When a listener indicates that he/she does not understand, the speaker's natural reaction is to repeat. If a single repetition works, it is a useful technique. When a second and a third repetition occur, with increasing tension and frustration, the chances for closing the circuit of communication go down.

A better technique is to rephrase the message. Try to make it shorter and simpler. In the doctor's office, for example, you may have whispered: "I guess we'd better sit down, Dad," and he failed to hear you. You can remedy the situation by turning so that he can see you, as you suggest: "Let's take a seat."

Speaking simply means using everyday vocabulary ("pay," rather than "remuneration") and short, direct sentences ("Bobby hit a home run," rather than "They said a home run was hit by our Bobby"). Sometimes wording the message like a telegram without complex grammar will make the point clear.

A special addition to rephrasing is reviving the context. This helps the hard-of-hearing person who needs a clue to the topic of conversation. "We were just talking about the ball game. Bobby's team played last night," are statements that revive the context and help orient. Oldsters who break in on a conversation they cannot really hear often jump to conclusions. Suspecting that people are making derogatory remarks, they become paranoid—quite unnecessarily.

To accommodate the aphasic persons you can edit your message in other ways. You can write it out if they seem unable to understand oral language, even though hearing is intact. Or you can point, gesture, or "act out" as you talk. It is best to present only one idea at a time and give enough time for a response before proceeding. Talk about present happenings and avoid abstract or controversial topics.

Barring other communication disabilities, neither the dysarthric patient nor the laryngectomee has any difficulty understanding language. There is no necessity for the speaker to edit either the length or the content of the message. As a courtesy, however, it is helpful to phrase questions so they require only "yes," "no," or a short answer. Since the dysarthric person moves the articulators with difficulty and the laryngectomee has trouble generating and sustaining a tone, brevity is a convenience. With astute listening and succinct comments they can play their role in the conversation with dignity.

Parodies vs. Parables

The dictionary defines a parody as a humorous, satirical, or burlesque imitation of a person, a composition, or an event. Parodies occur when we treat the elderly as less than real persons. In institutions, it is particularly easy to dehumanize, to stereotype, and to label the residents. During periods of illness, professionals and concerned family take over the patients' functions.

While victims may gain temporary status and attention by being ill, they can become gradually cemented in the quicksand of dependence. Knowing that they are no longer needed conflicts with the urge for rehabilitation.

Often the family proceeds to act a parody of their earlier life: Mr. X becomes the helpless dependent, while his son (or wife) acts as the authoritative, strong father. Roles are reversed and distorted. Someone else decides what he should eat, when he should sleep, where he should live. The anguish, shame, and frustration he feels only confound efforts to recover.

Even among the healthy elderly, family members may look for signs of "second childhood." Our culture has taught us to expect it. As muscle, sensory, and brain cells deteriorate, the elderly person often avoids the new experiences that would stimulate any residual powers. The family sees this withdrawal as a weakness and, in anticipation of a later dependence, acts as if that person is no longer a vital, contributing member of the group. Whether or not the intentions are good, making a parody of earlier family relationships does not promote the elderly person's self-mastery.

A better approach to an oldster who feels diminished is the use of parables, because they encourage independence. Like the short Bible stories, they use everyday people and events to convey a basic truth or moral lesson. They do not distort human relationships. They reveal positive "goods." They carry a special impact for the many oldsters who have refined their religious and philosophical ideas. What inspiration there is in the parable of the tiny mustard seed! An insignificant, apparently powerless, seed can yield a flourishing crop when it falls on fertile soil. What oldster does not hope that his/her remarks, advice, and insights will meet a receptive mind and yield a crop of pleasure, application, and understanding?

The use of parables allows the person to reverse condemnations, to see the bright side of life, to interpret events in ways that maintain mental health. For example, the necessary relinquishing of many personal possessions when an oldster moves to a retirement home can be seen as diminution of self or as a spreading of self and personal influence into the homes of family and friends.

"Your niece Kathy has asked for some of the Christmas tree ornaments, because she remembers what a happy time she had at your
home" is a more motivating remark than "They'll never let you take
all this stuff to the nursing home." Possessions can be interpreted
as having more value as gifts than as dust-collectors. The parable of
the rich man, "It is easier for a camel to go through the eye of a
needle than for a rich man to enter the Kingdom of Heaven," will
stimulate independence from objects and treasuring of personal
relationships instead.

SPECIAL ADAPTATIONS FOR THE INTELLECTUALLY
IMPAIRED

Undeniably, some oldsters do fit the description of senility—a decline
of mental faculties. They are forgetful, childish, and emotionally
labile. They have lost the ability to monitor or inhibit their behavior
and feel no embarrassment or shame. This last feature distinguishes
them from brain-damaged aphasics who may have laughing or crying
jags but feel frustrated and chagrined by their inability to control
them.

When communicating with someone who is genuinely demented,
simplify your message and allow plenty of time for a response. Give
only one direction at a time and demonstrate procedures. Avoid
lengthy explanations. When the patient wants to talk, use tactful
questions and reminders to maintain the general train of thought.
Showing intense interest stimulates the speaker's concentration and
can lead to longer, more meaningful exchanges.

The victims of intellectual degeneration experience confusion
and disorientation. They need to be reminded of the key features
of their present environment and daily schedule. "It's twelve o'clock,
time for lunch—in the big green room. That's the dining room."
They need to be reminded of who you are and, perhaps, of who
they are. Table 5.2 lists some of the most likely causes of dementia
and describes the associated speech/language symptoms. It includes
tips for management.

Parables, again, can be a good way of reinforcing a person's identity. These should be shortened parables that stress the everyday

TABLE 5.2   Communication Impairments Secondary to Dementia

Medical Case History	Speech-Language Symptoms	Management
Alzheimer's Disease (Progressive deterioration of memory, intellect, orientation, personality, and communicative functions—neural plaques and fibrillary tangles) Vascular or multi-infarct dementia From multiple strokes of TIA's or atherosclerosis (Diffuse cognitive losses) Parkinson's Disease— late stage (Tremor, masklike face, shuffling, and bent-over gait) Huntington's Disease Pick's Disease Chronic alcohol and/or drug abuse	• Jargon: bizarre content • Forgetting names or key words • Perseveration (involuntary repetition of words and phrases) • Speaking in sentence fragments • Expressing disjointed ideas • Circumlocution (talking around a subject) • Word meanings and social usages confused • Laughter or tears when not appropriate to the social context; little embarrassment or inhibition • Frequent topic shifting • Poor understanding of abstract or figurative language	• Repeat and remind patiently • Slow your rate of speaking and wait longer for a response • Increase demonstration and rehearsal of a task • Simplify explanations • Use a warm, nurturing vocal tone • Use singing and music to elevate moods • Notice the times and topics that stir a response • Don't argue with the "truth" of a statement; acknowledge with words that the person's feelings are "true" • Touch to stimulate; touch to reward; touch to "talk"

events and problems that you and the elderly person experience. They can be past events or current ones. They yield the double value of revealing you as a whole person and reminding the elderly person of his/her personhood.

Begin your abbreviated parable by finding the interests and experiences the two of you have in common. The old woman whose mind now wanders may have once been capable of managing a household and raising a family. Do you do that? Tell her. Make a little story about

TABLE 5.3 Summary Chart for Communicating Verbally With the Elderly Person/Disabled in Various Ways: How to Modify Your Speaking

For the hard-of-hearing:
    Speak louder, but do not shout.
    Articulate distinctly and visibly.
    Clue to the general topic.
    Rephrase specific and confused items.

For the receptive aphasic:
    Use common vocabulary, easy words.
    Speak slowly and distinctly.
    Use short, simple, direct sentences.

For the intellectually impaired:
    Remind them of time and place.
    Help them remember you because of a special trait.
    Use questions and tact to keep them on the topic.

a family event and share it. "My daughter has her first boyfriend. She feels so happy and flattered. This morning she got up extra early to iron her red blouse for school. It makes her look so pretty." Encourage her to tell about her first boyfriend, her daughter, or a red dress. Help her fix her clothes or hair.

The old man whose thoughts are scattered may have once been a plumber, a gardener, a Democrat, a sports fan. Which of his experiences can you relate to? Tell a story and try to get him to participate by asking his advice. "This year I decided to save on my food bills by planting a garden. The beans came up—and the lettuce and radishes. But I don't know what to plant in the shady part. What do you think?" Ask for instruction and explanation and report on the results. Keeping him apprised of the growth gives him a vicarious sense of accomplishment and a reminder of seasonal changes.

These abbreviated parables are not intended for philosophical discussion or drawing out of morals. The comparison to be made is between yourselves, as persons who play many roles in the past or in the present. The moral to be implied is that you both share a common humanity that cannot be destroyed by illness, institutions, or the adverse effects of aging.

See Table 5.3 for a summary of how to communicate verbally with elderly persons who are disabled in various ways.

MODIFYING YOUR LANGUAGE

The importance of using words both parties understand and of limiting the length and complexity of sentences applies to written language as well as oral language. Writing is a more permanent form than oral advice, and it can be read over as many times as necessary. Older folks who are aware of their memory lapses like to post notes as reminders, so written instructions give them a sense of security.

A group of beginning health professionals wanted to insure their accuracy in giving instructions. They hoped to get better compliance from patients by preparing a take-home packet of information in ways that circumvented the sensory and memory deficits of advanced age. They found the following modifications to be helpful.

1. Use large print in clear contrast to background. (Word processors offer fine choices of font, boldness, and size. But red ink on pink paper will not do.)
2. Use phonetic respellings of the necessary terminology. (The patients should be able to pronounce the words, so they will not be embarrassed to ask questions.)
3. Use no specialist definitions or equivalents of the terms.
4. Show uncomplicated diagrams, models, or photographs of required procedures.
5. Write medical information in a question/answer format or as a personalized memo.
6. Write post-treatment instructions or maintenance behaviors as a list of do's and don'ts.
7. List daily health procedures with check-off columns on a card to be posted on a refrigerator or bulletin board.

Language can be verbose or direct, dryly prescriptive or persuasive, memorable or forgettable. Your ability to spot the extremes in other people's remarks is surveyed at the end of this chapter, but your ability to monitor yourself must be practiced. Sensitivity to time, place, circumstances, and the message receiver is crucial. A true professional does not have to obfuscate or impress the client. Getting the message across is more satisfying than showing off.

TELEPHONING

Distance is a barrier to communication whether it is caused by family moves or the aged person's resettlement in a care facility. Since few of the oldest generation use e-mail, telephoning can be a good way to maintain contact without traveling. There are some recommendations that can make it more effective.

A recreation director reported on his family's long-distance telephoning problems:

> My grandmother only telephones for something very important—usually because she's in trouble. She's 80 now, and last summer she hit a tree when turning into the driveway. There were no injuries, but the car door was bashed in. I was on the extension phone and heard my own mother cross-examine like a cop and snappily give advice.
>
> Grandma was worried . . . should she give up driving, get the old (17 years) car fixed, or try to adjust to a new car? She didn't want to hear about taxis or the schedule of the senior bus.
>
> My mother's so cheap! She just wanted to get to the point, impose a solution, and get off the phone. Well, maybe she was anxious. When she's not around I just let grandma talk out her problems and ask what she thinks about various options. She makes her own decisions anyway. Matter of fact, she placed the call, at whatever expense, so it's her party.

The older and less affluent the persons are, the more likely they are to be nervous about long-distance calls. They often feel tongue-tied, because there is a charge for every minute. Nothing seems important enough to say, and the conversation falters. Such people feel more relaxed and pleased to get a letter—especially when it can be reread to a friend and enclosed snapshots can be shown around.

For those not inhibited by cost, timing is important, especially if the parties live in different time zones. Avoid meal times or rest periods. Even middle-aged children can feel bereft or worried if there is no answer, so it is a good idea to establish a mutually convenient schedule for calls. The seniors will feel pleased that their own social activities are recognized. For special occasions distant family and friends can arrange a conference call; everyone shares in the conviviality and takes turns talking.

Telephoning is a quick way to check on the mood and general health of oldsters who live alone. Until there are picture-phones the caller has just sound to tell "how well" the responder is actually feeling. But volunteers for Tele-Friend or Suicide Prevention testify that vocal quality gives voluminous cues. When video signals become part of phone transmission even more services will be possible—counseling, psychotherapy, remote diagnosis.

Speaking by phone to the hearing-impaired, aphasic, or disoriented person takes special patience. Use a medium-to-slow pace and pronounce words as clearly as possible. Aphasics should be asked to repeat the message in their own words to assure understanding. The intellectually degenerated listener misses not only the visual cues that aid communication but is taken by surprise out of his/her own train of thought. Be sure to identify yourself and explain the relationship and background of the message you want to share. To reduce misunderstandings a written confirmation of specific information (flight numbers, dates, times, etc.) should be provided as soon as possible thereafter.

Hard-of-hearing persons can have a desk-type phone modified to amplify incoming calls. For a modest price a receiver with a volume control dial can be attached, and its power range is greater than most hearing aids. Some oldsters will learn e-mail, and others, who are actually deaf, will use a teletypewriter (TTY) that plugs into a standard telephone jack.

TOUCHING

While telephone companies have urged us to "reach out and touch" someone, they did not mean it literally. But there are times when actually touching an older person facilitates communication more than anything else.

Touch, as a form of social interaction, is not popular in American culture—perhaps because it is such a vital part of sexual expression. But when physical and social welfare are seriously threatened, the preverbal basic need for firm, comforting touch surfaces.

Traditionally, nurses have the most societal permission for laying on of hands, because the daily caregiving activities—bathing, positioning, back rubs, changing dressings—all involve touch. Yet in geriatric care facilities, severely impaired clients are touched less than those who are mildly impaired. Furthermore, touch was utilized more often for instrumental (job-related) than for empathic (emotional) purposes. The philosophy of wholistic care would suggest that touch be used equally for both purposes.

Health care providers recognize that persons have different interpretations of personal space. Generally, the intimate zone is from the skin to 16 inches away. Professionals should ask permission before entering that zone, even doing a prescribed task (Schuster, 2000).

Many psychiatrists support the concept that healing touching serves as a corrective, emotional experience (Hutchison, 1999). A quick hug or a pat on the hand or shoulder can be a simple, positive reinforcement. Early diagnosis and treatment with generous praise and touch can even reverse symptoms of senility (Burnside, 1994).

A fine example of individual initiative is Jo Lindberg's hug therapy (Washburn, 1997). For many years she dressed up as Cuddles the bear and dispensed hugs to nursing home residents. In 1989 she set up the nonprofit Hugs for Health Foundation and vastly increased the number of volunteer huggers. She gives workshops to show how essential human touch is to a healthy life. The website is *www.hugs4health.org.* for students who believe hugs are good medicine.

The appropriateness of touch must be judged by the particular situation and the older individual's expressed or perceived need. For some, it might be interpreted as sexual, overly familiar, or a violation of personal space. But when there are signs of personal stress—tears, trembling—a gentle hand can do more than words to relieve the feelings of isolation and vulnerability.

EXERCISES

Language Awareness

The level of one's language should be appropriate for listeners. Please read the four remarks in each category and imagine for what audience they are appropriate. Then rate each on the scales from *verbose* to *direct, prescriptive* to *persuasive,* and so forth. For each of the four sets below, mark the items (a, b, c, d) at an appropriate place on the continuum.

Example:

Verbose   b, c...a, d   *Direct*
    a. Look at the person you're talking to.
    b. Considerate use of occulesics can help interviewees self disclose.
    c. Implement a systematic desensitization program for communication apprehension.
    d. Try to reduce stage fright.

1. *Forgettable*... *Memorable*
    a. Acculturation refers to the process of absorbing cultural traits by transference.
    b. As the twig is bent, so grows the tree.
    c. Vitamins won't improve your hearing.
    d. Vitamin C is contraindicated for cochlear degeneration.

2. *Prescriptive*... *Persuasive*
    a. You remember the "gipper," don't you? Ronald Reagan. Well, he wears his hearing aid all the time.
    b. I want you to cleanse the ear mold properly and keep it in for the full day. No cheating.
    c. Be sure to avoid enuresis; the aides resent it.
    d. After surgery a lot of people bed wet. Would you mind wearing this?

3. *Specialist's Jargon*... *Layman's Talk*
    a. Number 6 is edentulous.
    b. Mr. X isn't wearing his dentures.
    c. Termination of eligibility due to lack of documentation.
    d. Forgot to bring birth certificate.

4. *Pompous* .... *Practical*
    a. Mr. X is negatively disposed to civic affairs.
    b. He has a bad attitude to City Hall.
    c. Promulgate eligibility criteria for Title XX.
    d. Tell them about the meal program.

Other Exercises

1. Loudness can be monitored on the volume indicator (VU) meter of a tape recorder. Count to 10 raising your vocal power at each step. Holding your loudest tone, set the volume dial so the VU indicator peaks at 0. Keep the microphone at a uniform distance as you repeat rote phrases at various loudness levels.

2. Determine your speaking rate by reading aloud a passage of about 160 words and timing yourself. It should take a minute plus or minus a few seconds. Find another passage to read (from this textbook, perhaps), and underline the key words and phrases. Read it aloud giving greater duration to the meaningful phrases.

3. Check your ability to listen for information by watching a documentary show on television. Jot down the central thought and main points as you listen. Afterwards write a brief summary, and read it aloud to someone who viewed the same show. Listen to that person's evaluation, and weigh it against your own recall.

4. Here is a list of emotion-laden words. Mark with a plus sign those that arouse pleasant, positive emotions, and mark with a minus sign those that have negative connotations. Ask another person to mark the same list and explain any differences.

1.	Coronary	6.	Enterprise
2.	Prosperity	7.	Constipation
3.	Chocolate	8.	Snuggle
4.	Socialism	9.	Sneak
5.	Chauvinism	10.	Catharsis

5. Listen three times to a tape recording of adults with communication disorders. Listen once for what they say; listen twice for how they say it; listen finally to reinforce your memory and familiarity with the disorders.

REFERENCES

Burnside, I. (1994). *Working with older adults: group process and techniques.* Boston: Jones & Bartlett.

Hutchison, C. (1999). Healing touch: An energetic approach. *American Journal of Nursing, 99,* 43–48.

Schuster, P. (2000). *Communication: The key to the therapeutic relationship.* Philadelphia, PA: F. A. Davis.

Washburn, J. (1997). Hug therapy for seniors. *Good Housekeeping, 225,* 18.

6

Decision Making With the Elderly

At all stages in life there are decisions to be made. Choosing a partner, beginning or ending a career, handling money, and allocating leisure time are typical decision-making activities. As people age they become ever more aware of the limitations of time and energy, and the choices take on ever greater significance. The elderly must decide on a lifestyle commensurate with their health and resources. They are encouraged to name power of attorney, beneficiaries, even to purchase their own burial plot. And when the major decisions are made, such as a financial security plan and advance medical directives, there is a constellation of smaller choices—each day's economies in purchasing food, fuel, clothing, and so forth.

Decision making is a skill of adulthood. Only a young child, who acts before projecting consequences, can do it easily. If, with the addition of years, people also add knowledge, sensitivity to others, and experiences with the unpredictability of the future, then decision-making becomes more and more complex. As awareness increases so does the need to weigh and measure actions. To avoid legal and ethical problems, health care professionals press the patient and family to make end-of-life decisions (Stagno, 2000).

Within the family structure there are changes in the power of various members to influence decisions. Couples in the current generation may share power equally (egalitarian pattern), whereas older generations may reveal a conventional pattern of male dominance. As the young marriage ages the distribution of decision-making power may change, just as do the kind and quantity of decisions.

From an intergenerational sample of 315 Minnesota families, Hill and Mattessich (1987) found a number of changes in decision making over the life cycle of a family. The activities investigated were decisions about job change, moving, remodeling, redecorating, finances, and major purchases. The power in decision making showed an increase in wife-centeredness and a decrease in husband-centeredness and equalitarianism as age increased. Interviewers reported that authority seemed to reside with the wife in almost 20% of young marrieds but in up to 40% of grandparent families. The grandparent generation made the fewest plans, took the fewest actions, but fulfilled the highest proportion of its plans.

The process for rational decision making in families is not different from that used by business professionals (Kepner & Tregoe, 1981). It entails:

- identifying the problem
- discerning the necessary and the desirable features of its solution
- enumerating alternative means to the essential ends
- anticipating adverse consequences
- implementing the most attractive alternative

But in the Minnesota study where three generations were interviewed about decisions over the course of a year, the grandparents scored lowest on such steps. Young marrieds scored highest on the components of rationality, and middle-aged marrieds scored in the middle. The grandparent generation tended to rely on the immediate family as their only source of information.

Hence, those who are close to the elderly play a big part in decision making. You can assure that rational steps are followed if you slow down the process, amplify it, and make each step more graphic.

To help in the decision process you need to understand the psychological characteristics of elderly people in general and your elderly parent or patient in particular. For instance, as far back as Aristotle the elderly were characterized as conservative, inflexible, and philosophical in their view of life. Is that a true portrait of your friend? In what ways does your friend differ from this stereotype? How do these characteristics affect the ability to make decisions?

Current cultural stereotypes of patronizing, negating, and infantilizing the aged lowers their sense of personal control (Whitbourne, 1996). Health care situations are especially challenging. In cases of accident or acute illness the patient relinquishes control and accepts all dependencies. Weeks later he/she must be remotivated to take control again. As the most affected person the patient must share responsibility for diet regimens, health habits, and long-term rehabilitation.

You can help older persons by acting as a sounding board— reflecting and recording their thoughts as they work through the problem. If they skip a step, recall it to their attention. The following modifications to the decision-making process will make possible happier solutions and smoother transitions.

TIMING AND TACT

Often older people need more time to decide than younger people (Sliwinski & Buschke, 1999). The more serious the decision and the more commitment it entails, the more carefully it should be weighed. Periods of great emotional stress (death of a spouse or child) have to be worked through before logical thinking can occur. And that takes time. If deadlines tempt you to rush, be sure they are necessary deadlines, not mere bureaucratic conveniences. If the precipitating problem is not new, explore the possibility that it can be tolerated a bit longer. The adage about "acting in haste and repenting at leisure" can be devastatingly true, for instance, for someone who moves into an ill-chosen nursing home.

Tact is essential both in bringing up the problem and in defining it. Ownership of the problem must be clear. Age alone is no excuse for depriving a person of the right to make choices. Except for psychotic or long-term demented individuals, psychotherapy can stimulate decisional capacity (Frazer & Jongsma, 1999). The older people who are most content are those who made their own decisions regarding residence, finances, and social contacts. As an assistant, you can help by explaining the background of the problem and accepting any emotional outburst it calls forth. Anger, shame, and frustration can be explored. If the decision regards residence, key factors might be cost, convenience, and safety. The essential features of a solution need to be described, whether they are chosen by the person or imposed by the environment.

One of the first questions to be addressed is: On whom will the decision impact? (Noonan, 1999). From their past history and habits of responsibility the elderly often worry about family, friends, even grown children. Often they try to protect or overprotect those who no longer need their care. Any family ties need to be assessed realistically, and the independence of others can be tested in trial experiences or by recent history. Are the children finishing school, moving out, choosing mates? Maintenance of a large family homestead is not necessary if children are building their own homes or if they have not chosen to spend vacations at the homestead in recent years.

Another question to be raised is: What are the desirable features of a solution? These are the preferred but not essential elements. For instance, in deciding on a residence, the elderly person may *require* features like security, single floor, or proximity to a health clinic. He/she may *desire* features like a guest room, flower garden, or extra bathroom. By listing the desired features in order, you can be reminded of their relative importance.

EXPLORING ALTERNATIVES

All the many ways one could solve the problem need to be explored. What can we learn from expert advice, prior attempts, and/or personal experience? Are our assumptions valid? Do we have all the relevant facts? Are the facts from reliable sources?

Recording all the information on paper helps to clarify choices. The more complex the issue, the more confusion we experience. The very act of making a list organizes the mind and helps recall of details. Additions, new facts, and mental reservations should be written out too.

When change of residence is the task, taking a camera on each visit will give a record of what has been seen. Taking snapshots of the interior and exterior of the building as well as the surrounding neighborhood is a tremendous aid to memory when final decisions are to be made later.

Most decisions include objective elements (facts and figures) and subjective elements (personal attitudes and interpretations of the facts). Does a rundown neighborhood make you feel sad, unsuccessful, neglected, or discarded? The presence of subjective emotions in decision making cannot be denied, so bringing them out in the open is the sensible way of verifying their importance. Freud felt that if people followed their unconscious desires, they would experience deep well-being and psychic satisfaction. Writing out these factors in black and white helps us rate their actual value to our personal happiness.

CHARTING PROS AND CONS

Not only do the alternatives have to be amplified and explored in detail, but they need graphic representation in terms of preference. Any alternatives that do not meet the basic requirements of the solution can be eliminated. The others can be marked with stars to show how well they cover the desirable elements. Five stars, for example, could show the highest rating.

You can make a quick estimate if you have arranged the list of desirable elements in order of "most wanted" to "least wanted." Then, merely by seeing which alternative has the most stars near the top of the list, you see the most favorable choice. If the ratings are close, add up the number of stars. In Table 6.1, nursing home A would be the best choice, since all essential features are available and it has 6 more stars than home B in desirable features.

With the alternatives summed up, one might be tempted to act. But the elderly need time to adjust their thinking and to express their fears and reservations. This is totally valid. Even the best executives take time to imagine what adverse consequences there might be to a decision (Kepner & Iikubo, 1999). No matter how attractive the solution it may have disadvantages that are not immediately apparent. How will it impact on other conditions of life? What is its

TABLE 6.1 Choosing a Nursing Home

Essential Features	Home A	Home B
(*Must* have)		
State license	X	X
Moderate cost	X	X
(depends on individual's financial status)		
Physician on call	X	X
Skilled nursing	X	X
Fire safety	X	X
Cleanliness	X	X
Proximity to family	X	X
Secure building and grounds	X	X

Desirable Features		
(*May* have, in order of preference)		
Varied, well-prepared diet	****	**
Courteous staff	**	*
Speech Pathologist available	*	—
Physical Therapist	*	*
Private room	*	*
Grab bars in bathroom	*	*
Within 5 miles of son's residence	—	—
Activities programs	****	**
Catholic Church service	*	*
PREFERENCE TOTALS	15	9

Based on a guide from the American Health Care Association, Washington, DC.

future impact? How serious are the possible disadvantages? Are they real or imagined? How likely are they to happen?

During this period of reevaluation, paper and pencil are great helps. Again, write down the issues and rate them for their actual importance. The full chart of pros and cons should help focus discussion and enhance memory. Peruse the chart again and again until you both reach consensus. Consensus is not an enthusiastic "yes" vote, but rather a feeling of agreement. Even though some persons involved in the decision feel reluctance, when they reach consensus they are satisfied that the best of the available alternatives has been chosen.

MOBILIZING FROM PAST STRENGTHS

Plenty of lead time should be given prior to implementing a decision. Use that time to plan and prepare for as smooth a transition as possible; have detailed follow-up activities scheduled for the time period immediately after the change. The older people's faith is renewed when they see the evidence of your continuing interest and attention. It is the strength of your relationship that will help them over probable last minute waverings.

On the day of the change, the oldsters need to be well rested physically so there will be energy to absorb new impressions. Remind them of their residual power to control their own lives. Describe other instances in which they conquered fear and acted positively. Stay close as long as possible, and when you must leave, leave them with two simple chores to do. One of those chores must be reestablishing contact with you: "I'll be waiting for you to call me at 7." The other chore can be anything from scrubbing a sink to mailing a letter—any tie to the "here and now."

The older persons who are ill are the most difficult to mobilize, because they may have a generally pessimistic view of life. If they have passed through the stage of denying illness, they may be angry and resentful, looking for someone or something to blame. Or else depression and resignation to ill health may have led to self-pity and introversion. Rarely are the involuted ill sensitive to the needs of others. Having been stung so badly, they are afraid to change at all and become rigid in their behavior.

A logical approach is not sufficient to solve the problems of the ill, but arguments dealing with security and health will have a strong impact. The drive for self-preservation may still be strong. In an emotive approach, pleasant experiences can be associated with the change, and memories of past achievements should be revived: "This reminds me of the time you opened the shoe store on Brown Street. No one saw the potential of that location, but you stuck with it and made a profit." Or appeals to family pride can be helpful: "They didn't name you after Grandpa Hock for nothing; you're just as determined and brave."

Helping older people reach a decision is a humbling experience, not an ego trip. You have shared fears and hopes as they matched them against irrefutable facts of life. You reacted to emotions, re-flected ideas, reminded them of relevant steps, recorded the key factors, and reserved your judgment. The final decision was theirs.

EXERCISES

Deciding with the Elderly

1. Observe the behavior and thought processes of a consumer deciding on a clothing purchase. Does he/she enumerate alter-natives by trying on several garments? Does he/she proceed methodically? What desired features might lead to neglect of necessary features?
2. Find one or more real decisions that you or your friends face at present and write down a list of the necessary features of a solution. (In choosing a car, they might be price, mileage, seating capacity, etc.) Then make a list of desired features.
3. Your job is to select some young people to be trained as aides for a nursing home. What personal qualities would you look for, how would you set the standard for acceptance or rejection, and how would you measure the candidates against this stan-dard? Consider these elements:

Maturity level	Not overly helpful
Respectfulness	Grasp of nonverbal signals
Listening skills	Shows no favoritism
Relations with grandparents	Trustworthiness
Fear of catching illness	Cheerfulness

4. Role play the situation in which an offspring has to tell an aged person that he or she can no longer stay in his/her home. Begin with a complete description of the current situation and its drawbacks. After the older person is allowed to ventilate negative feelings, how is he/she drawn into generating solutions?
5. Often people will reach consensus because they place alterna-tives in the same rank order of value. Imagine Martha, newly

widowed and coping with arthritis, consulting her son and daughter. Should she sell the old house and go into an assisted living complex? The son ranks "safe" neighborhood far higher than "cleanliness." The daughter ranks having former "friends" among the residents far higher than physical therapy sessions. Will controversy between siblings inhibit Martha's choice? Try charting to resolve the problem.

REFERENCES

Frazer, D., & Jongsma, A. (1999). *The older adult psychotherapy treatment planner*. New York: John Wiley & Sons.

Hill, R., & Mattessich, P. (1987). Life cycle and family development. In H. Sussman & S. Steinmetz (Eds.), *Handbook of marriage and the family*. New York: Plenum.

Kepner, C. H., & Tregoc, B. B. (1981). *The new rational manager*. Princeton, NJ: Princeton Research Press.

Kepner, C. H., & Iikubo, H. (1999) *Managing beyond the ordinary* (computer file). Boulder, CO: netLibrary, Incorporated.

Noonan A. (1999). Getting to the point: Offspring caregivers and the nursing home decision. *Journal of Gerontological Social Work, 31,* 5–27.

Sliwinski, M., & Buschke, H. (1999). Cross-sectional and longitudinal relationships among age, cognition, and processing speed. *Psychology and Aging, 14,* 18–33.

Stagno, S. (2000). Bioethics: Communication and decision making in advanced disease. *Seminars in Oncology, 27,* 94–100.

Whitbourne, S. (1996). *The aging individual.* New York: Springer.

7

Group Involvement

In the life experience of most people, group participation is very common and beneficial. It touches a basic and elemental need of humans who are social animals. Very few people are complete "loners," and the majority are "joiners" of either formal or informal groups.

Since communication is a circular process, participants are most aware of themselves when they play an active role. In the situation where one person does most of the talking (as in teaching and preaching), we tend to hold that single person accountable for the message. In a dyad, or two-person communication situation (such as an interview), we hold both participants equally responsible. In a group situation, responsibility is spread thin and widely. We tend to feel free and toss out ideas and comments without much premeditation. We feel safety in numbers and may commit the group to levels of risk we would not undertake as individuals.

VALUES OF GROUP COMMUNICATION

For the elderly the primary value in being part of any group's workings is the lift in morale. They like to be consulted and know the inside information on prospective developments. They want to learn, to establish meaningful relationships, to relieve tension and worry, and to blend their attitudes and behaviors with those of the larger society. When they have had a reasonable opportunity to participate in problem-solving, they exert extra effort to make the solution work. Above all, they cherish the feeling of belonging.

In addition to being an excellent means for socializing, group discussion is a worthy method of learning. When no single member has complete knowledge of the topic, other members contribute their partial knowledge, so everyone reaches fuller understanding. Table 7.1 is an idealized balance of social and intellectual benefits though any particular group might emphasize either side.

The phenomenon of "group think" is one of the few known disadvantages of group communication. It occurs when more value is placed on bolstering group morale than on analyzing group tasks. Janis (2000) provides examples of government groups that have become victims of group think (for instance, President Kennedy's advisors for the Bay of Pigs invasion). Group members can become so loyal and eager to avoid conflict that they fail to scrutinize carefully the available courses of action. Some religious groups try to inspire deep economic sacrifices from their elderly adherents by using mass psychology slogans such as "join the bandwagon, . . . get on the Soul Train, . . . reserve your place in Paradise." Other groups like Families USA have rational leadership and broad enough membership (including all age groups) to avoid the pitfalls of "group think."

KINDS OF GROUPS

The first group that most of us experience is the family. In childhood, we receive many one-way messages from parents; in youth, we are more likely to engage in dialogue with parents. As our knowledge base equals or outdistances that of our parents we are consulted in general discussion of family enterprises for fun or general welfare.

TABLE 7.1 The Balance of Benefits

Clarifies thinking	Modifies attitudes
Supports self-efficacy	Stimulates problem-solving
Develops objectivity	Releases feelings and tension
Broadens interests	Reinforces belonging
Spreads information	Rehearses normative behavior

As middle-aged adults whose parents have moved out of the mainstream, we may regress to one-way communication again by either giving monologues of advice or receiving monologues of complaint.

When families are confronted with difficult decisions about the health, safety, and independence of older relatives, problems occur. How open or closed the family communication channels are influences the emotional costs paid by all concerned. Families that have a tradition of open discussion fare better and experience less stress.

Commonality groups are groups based on a shared interest, role, or status. Hobbyists may join to practice a particular art or craft. Sharing a particular employment category, church affiliation, ethnic status, or family role will give rise to relevant groups that cut across age boundaries.

Peer groups tend to consist of people of similar age as well as similar socioeconomic standing. In gerontology, the term *cohort* refers to age peers, that is, all persons born in the same year. Cohorts share the same historical era and perspective. The American Association of Retired Persons (AARP) is a peer group that lobbies for legislation benefiting all the aged. It is a good group for the older person who rejects purely recreational activity and still feels the need to be seriously involved in solving social ills.

Because most tax-funded programs for the elderly are administered by Parks and Recreation departments, there tends to be an emphasis on bingo, checkers, and leisure-time activities. Common interest groups become age-segregated, because grant givers set eligibility, accountability, and participation requirements. Small budgets and reliance on volunteers limit the range of interests that can be accommodated.

Most of the groups at a typical Senior Citizens Center are *socially-oriented,* that is, they meet for mutual encouragement and support. The conversation engaged in can take on the qualities of a discussion when it centers around a common problem or moves toward a common goal. But most often the communication patterns are informal. People move in and out of conversational clusters without threatening anyone's sense of belonging. They express opinions, insights, and experiences on random topics without feeling constrained by structured club rules and roles. What homogeneity exists comes from a shared interest in playing cards, folk dancing, oil painting, or other activities.

A *task-oriented* group functions for a specific purpose, such as fund-raising, neighborhood planning, religious indoctrination, self-governance, or any problem-solving activity. These groups have communication patterns that are more formally defined and structured than social or recreational groups. They have agendas, themes, leaders, and activities, all operating on a stated time schedule. Members of the group tend to become more alike in beliefs, attitudes, and behaviors the longer they stay with the group. This homogeneity contributes to the group's cohesiveness, or feeling of belonging. Members know each other's personalities and capabilities well enough not to set unreasonable expectations.

Although *cohesiveness* is a characteristic of an effective group, it cannot be forced. Pressure to conform can discourage members and drive away just the people who could originate novel means of reaching the group's goals. The older person who is perceived as cantankerous and critical may reveal a creative solution to a problem if granted a long enough interview. Genuine cohesiveness is based on respect for the individual. If one's loyalty is well known, that member can disagree and depart from the rules without suffering rejection. A fine example of cohesiveness is that among our legislators. Two congressional representatives can argue violently in a committee room, but, in the cafeteria, they return to solidarity.

Therapeutic Groups

Since the federal government reformed nursing home care in the late 1980s it has emphasized interdisciplinary therapy as a means to improve quality of care (Avery, 1997). These groups are designed to support the plan of care and involve nurses, psychologists, and social workers, as well as activity and recreation therapists. Ideally, these groups meet the needs of both short-term and long-term residents. All caregivers should be aware of the therapeutic methods and desired outcomes. Although it is difficult to measure objectively, staff members make a continual effort to observe behavior, to elicit feedback, and to record changes.

Groups open to the community at large usually have a self-selected membership, but those in residential institutions may be selected by the staff. In the latter situation, it is wise to interview prospective members to determine their attitudes and compatibility with other group members and the leader. Adding a blatantly negative person to a newly formed group can destroy its budding productivity.

Among therapy groups are those focused on reality orientation, reminiscing, and remotivation. Skilled leadership is particularly important in these groups, because the members generally view themselves as powerless to control their lives and effect changes in their environment. The leader must be supportive during and between meetings and must identify tasks that help the members develop some independence.

Reality orientation groups are designed for the institutionalized geriatric patient who is confused, disoriented, and suffering moderate to severe memory loss. Members meet regularly and the leader continually stimulates them with basic information—date, year, time of day, weather, next holiday, daily schedule, next meal, location of dining room, names of family, and other data. This procedure is intended to draw them out of isolation, increase self-care and self-direction, and restore contributing participation in the current environment. When patients are alert and fully oriented they know who they are, where they are, when things happen, and what their situation is.

Because the senses keep people in touch with the real world these programs often include sensory stimulation. The aged experience well-documented decrements in sight and hearing. Glasses and hearing aids are prescribed. But changes in the senses of taste, temperature, pain, and touch are less easy to measure and remediate. Activities that maintain the senses are helpful.

Validation therapy for residents with dementia was devised in the early 1980s by Naomi Feil. It is based on the humanistic tradition of psychotherapy and affirms that irrational speech and behavior occur for a reason. Validating what such persons say by encouraging and expanding messages shows unconditional regard for the individual who operates in a singular and distorted world. While reality orientation tries to draw the confused person into our world, validation therapy makes the client's world central to all verbal and nonverbal communication. Such empathic techniques can be delivered one-on-one or in groups. It has a calming effect and reduces agitation, aggression, and withdrawal.

There is logic in either approach, but little objective research into actual results. In 1997 (Toseland & Diehl) a study of 88 residents with dementia in four skilled care nursing homes compared validation therapy with social contact groups and a control group of usual care. The experiment lasted a full year. Nursing staff reported that members of the validation group were less physically and verbally aggressive and less depressed than members of the other two groups. But validation therapy was not effective in reducing use of psychotropic drugs and physical restraints.

A 1996 review of literature on the topic found that both reality orientation and validation therapy showed less promise than reminiscence groups. RO and VT failed to show adequate functional and psychological changes in clients to support the cost of implementation.

A *reminiscing group* allows members to explore the past. The value of such life review was first promulgated by Butler (1963). By returning past life to consciousness the older person reorders life, accepting what has been, and reevaluating the significance of those experiences. Sometimes old conflicts can be resolved and hasty judgments revoked. Memories can range from happy to somber, trivial to serious. Toseland (1995) cautions that remembering is not a form of rigidity or a way to avoid dealing with the present. The elderly use the past as a source of strength because their identity and self-esteem were formed at that time.

It is important for the group leader to show acceptance and appreciation. No matter how often the same event is recounted empathic listening must be maintained. Such repetition is not uncommon. Well-placed questions may draw out additional details or the reason for the strong emotional reaction and retention of that experience.

Remotivation therapy groups aim at reintegrating the institutionalized oldster into the current social world. Long-term, chronic patients may cling to symptoms because they are frightened of discharge. They need to become reinvolved in the world outside the institution, perhaps, even the world of work. Members are encouraged to communicate about past careers, current events, short poems, and news clippings. The group leader's special responsibility here is choosing compatible members who can compensate for each other. Alert, talkative patients need to be spread among members who are apathetic, fearful, or negative. The leader tries to enhance each one's image before the others so that the group's response will motivate further growth in sociability.

Support Groups

For the elderly with physical disabilities who are not institutionalized, support groups specific to their illness are very beneficial. People who have had cerebrovascular attacks can join a Stroke Club sponsored by the Heart Association or the Easter Seal Society. There are support groups for victims of Parkinson's disease, muscular sclerosis, cancer, alcoholism, overeating/self-starvation, and others. Hospice and Make Today Count try to meet the needs of those whose diseases are fatal. Such groups help educate the members and the public, build morale, and provide a halfway experience before reintegration into other community groups. Sometimes the groups raise funds for research and prevention of the special condition.

The phenomenon of self-help groups has grown enormously over the past several years. The Public Health Service estimates that 18 million people in the United States have banded together in half a million groups designed to help members face the crucial challenges of life, such as divorce, illness, addiction, child-rearing, job loss, disability, and death. The idea has become so popular that there are at least 24 regional clearing houses have been set up around the country to help troubled callers find the appropriate organization.

The criteria for joining a specific support, self-help, or mutual aid group is not age. It is sharing a similar problem or shattering experience. While anorexia nervosa is generally considered to be a teenager's or a young woman's problem, it happens to oldsters too. The motives are different. It is not likely to be a conscious choice for the elderly, but a happenstance, a gradual slipping away from life. There is less incentive to cook when there is no family around, or taste buds seem dormant, or bland diets are required, or the prospect of cleaning up looks overwhelming. The half-hearted cook can forget food is on the stove and face unappetizing, burned, or dried out meals. Glamour is not an issue, but survival is.

Anorexia Is Ageless

A human services trainee reported on her neighbor Celeste L: Celeste was a farmer's wife living down a long, lonely lane. In her sixties, she became severely arthritic and depended thoroughly on her husband and a family doctor several years older than she. The physician's death, when it came, was not untimely, but it stopped Celeste's clock. She lost interest in living. Feeling lost and abandoned, she had no incentive to eat or keep up her strength. Always tiny, she lost weight dramatically.

From a farm family herself, the trainee stopped over with casseroles or baked goods from time to time, but the worried husband was the only one who relished them. Celeste became white-haired and fragile as a bird. She appeared more spindly than a dove, but just as peaceful. When her husband died Celeste moved into town, and the increase in daily exercise required to manage the household alone stimulated her appetite. Her new neighbors got her involved in the Meals on Wheels program. The self-imposed anorexia was not totally turned around, but Celeste ate enough to sustain herself for another 8 years.

PROCEDURES IN GROUPS

The procedures in a *task-oriented* discussion are directed toward reaching the group's goal. Participants seem to proceed in spurts of energy, but the discussion is not random. Fisher (1994) describes the activity in four phases:

Phase 1: Orientation—Getting acquainted, clarifying, and tentatively expressing attitudes.

Phase 2: Conflict—Disputing, dissenting, controversy, conflict. Members leave the tentative stage and begin to make up their minds.

Phase 3: Emergence—Dispute, dissent, conflict begin to dissipate. Members whose point of view is beginning to lose out retreat from their firm positions by making ambiguous statements. The eventual outcome of the discussion is beginning to emerge.

Phase 4: Reinforcement—Argument no longer seems important. Comments favoring the emerging outcome are reinforced.

In *socially oriented* groups, there is a less-structured procedure, but not the randomness of casual conversation. The steps are as follows:

1. Suggesting a timely or important topic: "How did Labor Day get started? What types of jobs are organized into unions?"

2. Generating ideas and questions about the topic: "Commercial or mechanical work doesn't require acreage. What are disadvantages of farming?"
3. Regulating participation so all members have an equal chance in a climate of mutual respect: "As Bob was saying." "Good point." "And what do you think, Bill?"
4. Refocusing the discussion when the mood or comments of the participants wander too far from the topic: "Every occupation requires special skills. What are the skills for factory work? Have any of you tried it?"
5. Pointing out relationships between statements made by different persons at different times during the discussion: "That reminds me of what Agnes said." "Doesn't that support Jim's first point on skills?"
6. Closing the discussion with a concise summary of the principal contributions: "Labor Day commemorates the workers' movement toward greater recognition of their skills and commitment."

FUNCTIONAL ROLES

The concept of role is borrowed from the theatre. Just as an actor is chosen to portray a character in a play, so we are guided by society to act in certain ways. A script tells the actor how to behave in relation to other characters. We are guided by education and our own sensitivity to social pressure. Any individual plays a variety of roles in daily life, depending on the time, the place, and the situation. If all the members of a small group accept some role responsibilities, goals can be reached with a minimum of confusion.

Here are some member roles that facilitate task-oriented behavior:

1. Contributor—gives information and opinion
2. Clarifier—explains issues and situation as whole
3. Harmonizer—looks for commonality, resolves conflict
4. Orienter—gives a reality check to ideas and actions

As a group grows in size and structure the tendency is to choose a leader to act as manager and spokesperson. The role is a mixed blessing, but it is a measure of the person's trustworthiness. Patience and tolerance are also prized if the group has a high proportion of elderly people.

Leadership in self-help groups can be given by peers or trained professionals. In a detailed study of the Supportive Older Women's Network (SOWN), Kaye (1997) found that members in peer-led groups experienced the greatest gain in emotional support and increased social networks. Members in professionally led groups experienced more gain in the instrumental domain. They could legitimize their concerns, find technical information and link to other social services. To blend benefits, peer leaders sought out training in facilitation and professionals appeared as guest informants.

In a national study of group work in skilled nursing facilities (Mazza & Vinton, 1999), the majority offered both educational and support groups for residents and for family members. The typical leaders were social service staff (60% of whom had social work degrees).

Burnside (1994) recommends that leaders of the frail elderly have the ability to handle their own feelings regarding chronic illness, disabilities, depression, grief, hostility, and the various stages of dying. Somehow leaders meet these challenges day after day with a smiling face and a soothing voice.

MAINTAINING GOOD PARTICIPATION

What keeps a group alive is its membership. There must be rewards of some kind entailed with belonging to the group, or individuals will return to their own affairs. In the most authoritarian group, the autocratic leader dispenses bits of power and prestige to followers. Even the least influential member can feel rewarded by association and identification with the strength of the organization. In socially oriented groups where there is less power and more permissive leaders, members are rewarded by the supportive, relaxing social interplay.

Among service providers to the elderly there is growing recognition of the need for group discussion and participation as a means of increasing knowledge, stimulating personal growth, and exchanging experiences. Although the healthy, independent older person may participate in powerful, task-oriented groups that deal with substantive issues like politics or economics, the ill rarely do. Some nursing homes do have groups for self-governance, but their powers are fairly limited.

Poor health not only reduces one's ability to take responsibility, but also reduces inhibitions. The ill resident may talk too much or too irrationally or express such bitterness and negativism that others are discouraged from returning to the group. For such reasons it is wise to set some rules for courtesy:

- Concentrate on the content of what others say.
- Welcome any new ideas; poor ideas will collapse without reinforcement.
- Make no negative remarks about other people's contributions.
- Avoid judging the motives of others.
- Avoid interrupting whenever possible.

Often the vision and hearing deficits of the elderly make it difficult to know when someone is still talking or is trying to break into the repartee. What seems to be rude, insensitive behavior is merely poor sensory input. Try rearranging the seating—use a circle or semicircle so that vision can supplement hearing.

The behaviors of each individual in a group can be observed objectively to show progress in socialization. You can make a very simple analysis by checking the number of times each member spoke. This basic counting technique allows you to see who are the active or inactive communicators in this specific group. More information is gleaned by tabulating the kinds of communicative acts, such as asking questions, making statements, supporting others or rejecting ideas. A group of four people making Christmas ornaments can be charted as shown in Table 7.2. By observation, D is silent and C talks most; B and C seem to share a lot.

The responsibility for maintaining good participation rests, in part, on the leaders. Generally, democratic leaders are willing to be a part of the group and to let others take the spotlight. With patience and empathy, they can build up the confidence of reluctant oldsters to the point where they end up contributing. Because members feel

TABLE 7.2 Objectifying Communicative Acts in a Small Group

Participant	Asks questions Seeks advice	Makes statements Gives advice	Rejects ideas	Supports others
A	1	1	1	0
B	1	11	0	1
C	11	1111	0	1
D	0	0	0	0

greater faith, security, and self-confidence, they keep coming back to the group.

SUGGESTED TOPICS FOR DISCUSSION

Any topic that is of general concern to older people is a topic for discussion. Within the family, common subjects are food, health, clothing, shelter, attitudes, and morale. The same topics occur in age-related community groups. For instance, a Senior Citizens Forum might deal with nutrition, investment and income planning, alternative housing, and positive thinking. Church and non-age-segregated community groups (such as political parties) tend to deal with the same topics perennially, but the input of the older person varies with his/her deepening insights. In the social hour that comes before or after the business meeting, casual conversation can be highly varied.

Talking about one's occupational roles and experiences is a natural and popular topic with the elderly. The routines and work methods of factory, office, farm, and household can be described with much detail. Such reminiscences of one's productive period build identification and self-esteem. When people have known the person for a long time there is less room for exaggeration, but in retirement villages making new friends often entails "gilding the lily," a harmless puffing up of past successes.

Giving advice makes a rousing discussion. The advice can be in the form of directions (how to refinish old furniture) or problem-solving. The latter occurs when controversial political or personal affairs have occurred, and second-guessing is rampant. Such as "In spite of the polls Truman carried our state in the 1946 election," or "We like our neighbors but their yard is a shame—crabgrass junk!" Newspaper columns like "Dear Abby" stimulate the exchange of opinions and parallel experiences.

The elderly who are ill and confined to a nursing home may feel a shrinking of horizons. The recreation director or occupational therapist makes an effort to learn about the residents' past occupations and interests so they can be included in discussions.

Seasonal topics are particularly helpful in maintaining reality orientation; so are physical chores. An accompanying activity, like tree-decorating at Christmas or apple-peeling and pie-making in the autumn, arouses many mental associations and pleasant memories. Any simple activity that serves a useful purpose raises the self-esteem of participants too. They are likely to talk more and the topics they bring up should be recognized by the leader and explored with the rest of the group. Well-phrased questions can keep attention on the topic until everyone has voiced an opinion or insight. The leader in a nursing home environment values the *process* of discussion just as much, if not more, than the *product* of discussion.

EXERCISES

1. Take part in a class discussion and count the number of negative remarks made. Observe their effect on the people to whom they were addressed. Did criticism tend to stimulate or inhibit contributions?

2. Listen and watch a televised discussion of current affairs. How did the leader introduce the topic and explain the procedure? Rate the leader on the following functions:

	Inadequate	Adequate	Good
Starting the discussion			
Engaging the participants			
Maintaining balance among participants			
Making transitions to new material			
Acknowledging responses			
Coping with controversy			
Summarizing			

3. Select a classic theme, such as "Love conquers all barriers" or "Cheaters never prosper," and start a small group discussion. Ask two people to act as observers. After 15 minutes have the observers rate the participants:

	Inadequate	Adequate	Good
Awareness of others			
Deference to leader			
Listening empathically			
Speaking clearly and concisely			
Clearing up ambiguities in meanings			
Sticking to the subject			

4. With a small group, role-play a situation, such as counseling a bereaved widow or persuading people to donate funds to a church or charity. Follow the role play with a discussion (what approaches and persuasions were omitted, what were extenuating circumstances?). Tabulate the kinds of communicative acts that occur for one individual. Use the chart presented in the section Maintaining Good Participation.

REFERENCES

Avery, L. (1997). *Activity programming in long-term care.* New York: Springer.

Butler, R. (1963). The life review: An interpretation of reminiscence in the aged. *Psychiatry, 26,* 65–76.

Burnside, I. (1994). Leadership and co-leadership issues. In I. Burnside & M. Schmidt (Eds.), *Working with older adults: Group process and techniques* (3rd ed.). Boston, MA: Jones & Bartlett.

Fisher, B. A. (1994). *Small group decision making: Communication and the group process.* New York: McGraw-Hill.

Janis, I. L. (2000). Victims of group think: A psychological study of foreign policy decisions and fiascoes. In D. Barash (Ed.), *Approaches to peace.* New York: Oxford University Press.

Kaye, L. (1997). *Self-help support groups for older women.* Washington, DC: Taylor & Francis.

Mazza, N., & Vinton, L. (1999). A nationwide study of group work in nursing homes. *Activities, Adaptation & Aging, 24,* 61–73.

Toseland, R., & Diehl, M. (1997). The impact of validation group therapy on nursing home residents with dementia. *Journal of Applied Gerontology, 16,* 31–51.

Toseland, R. (1995). *Group work with the elderly and family caregivers.* New York: Springer.

8

Promoting Self-Expression

Among the psychological changes associated with aging, there is a tendency is to withdraw and become relatively more introverted, whatever the earlier personality charactcristics were. For some individuals disengagement leads to meditation and inner peace, but for many it means loneliness and depression. An obvious solution is to provide many opportunitics for social contact and self-expression and yet allow individuals to reject or adopt them by their own choice.

Considering that there are two main personality types in the general population, we can offer activities that suit both. For extrovert types, oral communication is a way of venting feelings and maintaining social contact with present companions. For introvert types, written communication is a way of venting feelings and maintaining social contacts with people who are distant in place or time. Each type of communication is satisfying because it assumes a human response—a listener or a reader—and while oral communication is usually a victim of the "here and now," it can be audio- or video-taped and played back to distant friends and later generations.

Although all artistic endeavors allow self-expression, music and art will not be discussed in this chapter. The wide range of arts and crafts shows and concerts are evidence that these diversions are already well-organized and readily available. The creative uses of language are more likely to be ignored, because the product is not as easily observed and comprehended.

Yet creative communication can yield not only social and emotional benefits but also enhanced mental activity. A cardiologist who still runs marathons in his sixties claims, "The way to improve thinking is through expression. If you don't sing or write you don't know what you think." His mind and body are almost separate when he runs, and he uses the time to write his medical column for a sports magazine in his head.

FACTORS IN MOTIVATION

The elderly ill are the most likely to lack motivation for communicative self-expression. For them, disengagement may mean losing touch with other people altogether. Stroke victims, for instance, frequently testify to the feeling of isolation and claim that their recovery was due to motivation as well as therapy.

Although the factors in motivation have been understood intuitively, making a list of them increases the awareness of all the participants in the rehabilitation process. This would include doctors, nurses, aides, and therapists of all types. They need to know the conditions that stimulate patients' active interest in their own rehabilitation.

There are many theories of motivation (e.g., cognitive, associative), but the humanistic theory is most concerned with explanations of mature adult behavior. It is based on naturalistic observations of people as well as in-depth interviews.

Of the several theories that can be described as humanistic, Abraham H. Maslow's theory stands out as the most clearly motivational. He posits a hierarchy of seven sets of needs. They include (1) physiological, (2) safety, (3) belongingness and love, (4) esteem, (5) self-actualization, (6) desires to know and understand, and (7) aesthetic. The higher order needs can be manifested only after needs lower in the hierarchy have been satisfied.

Patients with a neurological impairment or degeneration may feel threatened at any or all of these levels. They must be compensated for any deficits in areas 1 and 2 because they concern survival. In area 3, belongingness and love, they can be seriously affected by loss or desertion of a marriage partner or family members. With increasing age and loss of employment, the patient can be deprived in area 4. Since the patient is unable to fulfill lower level needs, it is highly unlikely that self-actualization or any of the needs beyond it will bc attained.

ESTABLISHING A CONDUCIVE ENVIRONMENT

Some conditions must be met for self-expression with language. They are privacy, quiet, and respect. The right to privacy encompasses choice of associates and must be interpreted reasonably. When a loved companion dies or when one is consigned to a health facility, the favored choices may not be possible. But in the simplest of daily activities there are possibilities for choice, and such freedom must be protected. The need for quiet is obvious whenever someone tries to write a letter or carry on a meaningful conversation in the same room with a loud television. The need for respect is violated when outsiders look at someone's diary or mail without permission. Respect entails making space for souvenirs, old photo albums, artifacts, and mementos.

A conducive environment also offers rewards for self-expression. All of us want our remarks listened to, our jokes laughed at, our letters answered, and our complaints commiserated with, if not solved. The two-way nature of communication must always be maintained, although differential amounts of attention are paid depending on the life-adjustment value of the expression. For instance, time consuming as it is, reading someone's life history will lead that person to further writing and exploration. In oral communication, a high-level reward occurs when suggestions from an individual or group are actually implemented.

In institutions for the elderly, discussion groups can be organized, talking rooms or coffee corners set aside, and mealtimes modified for socialization. The British have a gracious system: coffee in the drawing room. It was conceived as a convenience for the staff. Dinner being completed, clean-up can be carried on while the residents follow a tea cart to a social room. The camaraderie and relaxation brought on by a warm meal are transferred to another location. No one is rushed. The staff members clean up the coffee cart the next morning.

Suggested Activities for Oral Communication

1. Encourage and reward all "I" statements. Such revelations of the person's feelings, fears, angers, and so forth are more manageable when not repressed. Otherwise bitterness, frustration, sulking, and volcanic explosions can occur. Language can ameliorate the darkest emotions.

2. Develop a bargaining philosophy. Guide your elderly friend through the process of discovering what he/she really wants and what he/she is willing to give. Show how necessary tradeoffs can lead to a happier life. Exploring a situation from two different standpoints also reinforces the maturity needed to reverse condemnations. Instead of saying "My son is selfish; he never comes to see me," the complaint can be reversed, "I wish I'd been more cheerful and entertaining the last time he came, so he'd feel like visiting sooner."

3. Encourage a problem-solving attitude by discussing a favorite TV show after each showing. Discuss the crises, their causes, the relevant characters, and the next most likely event. This activity exercises memory, logic, and imagination.

Additional Activities for Group Living

1. Make space for a quiet talking room or "chat" corner. At parties or special dinners arrange the seating plan to mix "talkers" and "nontalkers."

2. Establish a discussion group, advisory council, hobby group, or Toastmaster's Club. These groups use speech as a tool. The activities are goal-oriented and self-perpetuating.

3. Arrange get-acquainted parties or a talent show where staff and patients can be seen in three dimensions, not merely in stereotyped roles.

ADVANTAGES OF THE LIFE REVIEW

The elderly have a strong interest in summing up. Those who are emotionally healthy and alert engage in an active, or purposeful, examination of the events of their lives so as to leave behind an acceptable image.

Butler (Butler, Lewis, & Sunderland, 1998) claims that a life review can enhance the quality of retirement years. Reviewing the past, by writing it out, helps to resolve conflicts and regrets. It helps to reconcile personal relationships. One writer, for instance, upon re-examining events, forgave a former business partner against whom he had held a grudge for almost a decade. In summing up one's life work, it is possible to gain insights into one's purposes and integrate them into the present and the future.

Haight (1992) examined the long-term effects of a structured life review. The persons involved increased their life satisfaction and well-being for as long as twelve months. In England similar programs show that telling the life story can have "tremendous effects on well-being" (Viney, 1993).

Retirement is the ideal time for personal memoirs, because one has gained the wisdom of experience and the time to reflect. When he was 80, Johann Wolfgang Goethe was asked to reissue his poems with his own critical interpretations. His reply was:

> At that period of life when knowledge is more perfect and conscious-ness most distinct, it is a very agreeable and reanimating task to treat former creations as new matter and work them up into a kind of Last Part.

AUDIO/VIDEO TAPING FOR POSTERITY

Audiotaping memories is a popular way of reviewing one's life. As it creates a historical record of a person, it also shows the cultural milieu, and historians value such data. To fully understand an era and a particular community, historians need the testimony of ordinary people, as well as the written records of politicians and celebrities. One of the most extensive collections of interview data is held by the U.S. Holocaust Memorial Museum (1998).

At the same time as oral history has won acceptance as a legitimate academic pursuit, it has found its way into entertainment. In television documentaries, there has been a shift away from interviews with famous people toward interviews with the non-elite. Reporters encourage people to tell their story as a shortcut to interpreting historical events. If the speaker rambles, the tape is cut and edited to keep only the parts relevant to the producer's goal. Such activity might lead to legal and ethical challenges of misrepresenting the resource person. To protect against abuses, interviewers use a consent form that details the purpose, the dissemination, and the possible editing of the tape.

For a private, personal oral history the tape should only be edited for topical or chronological sequence. A good interviewer can guide the testimony to follow particular themes.

- What was your relationship with your parents?
- With your children?
- What are your feelings about the United States in the twentieth century?
- About politics past and present?
- What are your views on the physical life, love, marriage, sex, religion, travel, work, and retirement?
- How do you feel about grief and death?

Videotaping is certainly more expensive than audio recording, but it preserves visual data and is much more likely to be reviewed. Many homes have video equipment already, so as cameras and tapes come down in price more families will be able to keep a record of loved ones—young and old.

Preplanning can prevent long pauses and disorganization. If the speaker makes notes of key words, dates, and names and a partner develops follow-up questions, the filming will move at a good pace. The machine can be stopped at intervals to allow for rehearsal, reflection, and/or organization, or the final tape can be edited to remove awkward pauses.

WRITING FOR POSTERITY

Writing one's reminiscences is an inexpensive pastime. It allows the older person to conquer time and gain the keen pleasure of mental stimulation and ego involvement.

The life review can be started with just a scrapbook of old newspaper clippings and souvenirs or a family album. Writing titles for each page and captions for the pictures stimulates memory. Listening to old phonograph records at the same time can revivify moods of the past.

Keeping a diary or journal is another good step toward writing a personal history. The main advantage is getting into the habit of writing down experiences on a regular schedule. Furthermore, the writer tends to view events in perspective and make sense of them in the recording process.

Generally, there is a distinction between a diary and a journal. The first is a day-to-day record of daily events, whereas a journal is a record of intellectual and spiritual growth. The definitions overlap. A diarist may interpret events in a way that reveals personal beliefs and general philosophy. A journalist may tie general reflections on life to the memory of specific events. People from all walks of life have enrolled in journal workshops. They seek self-actualization and refinement of the self-concept (Adams, 1998). They don't need therapy, but they want to put their lives in perspective.

For a writer the greatest resource is memory. It is mined to assemble as much usable material as possible. No pick or shovel is needed, just concentration. Whole events can be relived by the process of association, that is, linking images, sounds, and ideas to create a full mental picture of the past. These clusters of recollection are the necessary background for telling a story.

Memory and artistry work together in drawing the foreground. The vivid and meaningful elements of one's mental picture are delineated with enough detail to enlighten the reader. Great masses of encyclopedic detail would overwhelm the reader, so they are deleted. They rest in the back of the mind, helping the writer choose the few, choice words that convey a mood.

It is just this reality of a reader that makes writing a personal history such a stimulating adventure. Although writing may seem like a monologue, it is actually a dialogue with a silent partner—the reader. The writer imagines a person of intelligence and goodwill whose mental questions are answered with as much explanation as necessary.

Often a person has experienced a life-changing event—natural disaster, war, famine—where the outside world must be described.

Tom Brokaw (1998) felt that the defining event of the 20th century was World War II. He interviewed members of that generation to get a full view of that major event. In relating events of the First World War, women had to see the event from the establishment's point of view as well as their own (Cardinal, 1999). Whether the story is about inner, private life or outer, public life it must be organized well enough for an outsider to understand it.

Here are some basic organizational plans:

1. Time: Maintain a chronological pattern beginning at a certain period and moving forward: "My Americanization began when the boat docked at Ellis Island in 1927."
2. Cause-effect: Tell what the precipitating factors were and what results they have had: "If I had not become a teacher, I wouldn't have become involved in the first, original teachers' strike."
3. Personal/general: Explain how the events affected you personally and then how they affected others or society in general: "The hurricane of 1955 not only ripped off my home and office, it divested the Milford community of thousands of dollars."

Only the most accomplished writers can plunge in without an organizational plan. Mark Twain, the United States' humorist, wrote an autobiography that resembled a series of entertaining dinner table talks. He recommended the "methodless method of the human mind," and he described it like this:

> Start at no particular time of your life; talk only about the things which interest you for the moment; drop it the moment its interest threatens to pale, and turn your talk upon the new and more interesting thing that has intruded itself into your mind meantime. (Twain, 1959, p. xi)

The sustained mental effort of writing long pieces is usually not possible for the elderly ill. But Koch (1999) demonstrated that nursing home residents found pleasure in writing short poems. His program was structured to draw out poetic expressions rather than formally crafted sonnets. Every contribution was read aloud and praised for its poetic elements (strong emotion, comparisons, imagery, sensuous detail, repetition), not for rhyme patterns or metrics.

Patients who were unschooled, depressed, or dying all responded, and when they lacked strength to handle pen and paper, volunteers took dictation.

Such devotion to creative writing seems unbelievable, until it is experienced. The work can go on anywhere—a doctor's office, a hospital, at Hospice—as the writer makes a mental leap to a different level of existence (Bolton, 1999).

EXERCISES

Suggested Activities for the Writer

There are particular advantages to setting up a writers' group at a senior center or residential facility. Little or no equipment or supplies are needed. A single staff member or volunteer can handle any size group without additional training. The activity extends far beyond the actual hours of face-to-face contact.

The following are typical activities for club members:

1. Keep contact by writing letters. Make a list of your distant readers' hobbies and personality characteristics. Stress the two-way nature of communication by asking for their comments and advice. Leave a pleasant impression by telling them a joke on paper.
2. Haiku is a form of poetry originated by the Japanese in the 14th century. Each word or phrase conjures up an image or train of thought. The form is three lines: first line is five syllables long, second is seven syllables, and third is five syllables. Prepare two haiku for sharing.
3. Describe a city block, street, or particular neighborhood in your town that has changed in noticeable ways. Choose an area changed by new buildings, commercialization, fire, and so forth. Make a clear contrast between what it was and what it is now.
4. Begin a diary by considering the elements of "newsmaking." Write headlines for daily events and tell who, what, when, and

where. Analyze the "why" when you are in a reflective mood and put that reasoning in a journal.

5. Explore your roots and flesh out the family tree by writing personality sketches of your favorite relatives. Find your place in major historical events by writing eyewitness accounts. Describing the personal impact of events may lead to longer works for which you choose an organizational plan.

Additional Activities for Group Living

1. Enlist volunteers to read or to interview those who want to leave a permanent record of their life's events.
2. Invite a local university or library to make an oral history investigation of public crises and their impact on individuals in the local community.
3. Practice some "old fashioned ways," like shucking corn or peeling apples, and tape-record the memories they stir. Later review the tape and use it as a stimulus for further self-expression on paper.
4. Enlist local actors or volunteers to read aloud. They can prepare excerpts from popular personal writing, such as J. Durrell's *Beasts in My Bed*, B. Magione's *An Ethnic at Large*, Tom Brokaw's *The Greatest Generation Speaks: Letters and Reflections*, or Ben Franklin's autobiography.

REFERENCES

Adams, K. (1998). *The way of the journal.* Lutherville, MD: Sidran Press.

Bolton, G. (1999). *The therapeutic potential of creative writing.* Philadelphia, PA: Jessica Kingsley.

Brokaw, T. (1998). *The greatest generation.* New York: Random House.

Brokaw, T. (1999). *The greatest generation speaks: Letters and reflections.* New York: Random House.

Butler, R., Lewis, M., & Sunderland, T. (1998). *Aging and mental health.* Boston: Allyn & Bacon.

Cardinal, A. (Ed.). (1999). *Women's writing on the First World War.* New York: Oxford University Press.

Haight, A. (1992). Long-term effects of a structured life review process. *Journals of Gerontology, 47,* 312–315.

Koch, K. (1999). *Learning by heart.* Iowa City, IA: University of Iowa Press.

Twain, M. (1959). *Autobiography of Mark Twain.* Edited and with an introduction by Charles Neider. New York: Harper Brothers.

U.S. Holocaust Memorial Museum (1998). *Oral history interview guidelines.* Washington, DC: Author.

Viney, L. *Life stories: Personal construct therapy with the elderly.* Chichester, England: John Wiley & Sons.

9

Computers and the Oldest Generation

When computers first caught public attention they were seen as miracle calculators operated by highly intelligent people using arcane codes. When children began to use them for games and instruction (as schools acquired hardware and software) middle-agers became curious. Then development of the personal computer with friendly user interfaces and competitive pricing brought about widespread acceptance.

Now over half of all American families own a PC. While about 25% of people over age 60 have a computer (often a hand-me-down from fully employed sons or daughters), more than one-third ranked PC's as "only slightly useful." They find the device difficult to use (McConnaughey, 1998). Yet it is today's premier tool for expressive (writing) and receptive (reading) communication.

At retirement aging baby boomers will already be computer savvy and have their favorite uses—communication, information, shopping, stock-watching, entertainment, or socializing. As they experience increasing deficits in vision, hearing, speech, mobility, or coordination, the industry will develop ever more ways to circumvent such losses. Even now voice-operated systems are in place, such as voice-enabled e-mail. The Rehabilitative Center for Adapted Technology (RECAT) in Scottsdale, AZ trains the disabled so that even the slightest movement (a blink or glance) can operate the computer. Prentke Romich already publishes a complete manual about obtaining funds for compensatory devices from Medicare, Medicaid,

Vocational Rehabilitation, Veterans' Administration, and others (Romich, 2000).

But what about the oldest generation? How can they benefit? In 1998 the National Telecommunications and Information Administration set a goal to connect all Americans to the Information Superhighway. As expected, seniors showed low participation—only 8% had on-line access to the Internet. Other have-not categories were low income, low education, minorities, and rural residents. The U.S. Census Bureau cross-tabulated data for the three preceding years and found that PC ownership had increased 52%, modem ownership, 139%, and e-mail access, 397% (McConnaughey, 1998). The last figure is especially significant because e-mail is the favorite choice of the older persons who do use computers. If Internet access were also free and fast they might use it more.

Policymakers urged schools, libraries, and community access centers to help the "least connected." This works best when there is full time assistance available because older learners get as frustrated as anyone else when a search for information goes in circles. While students and working people use library computers on a predictable schedule, elders fill in during the slack hours. Gracious and patient librarians have played an important role in conquering the digital divide.

There have been numerous projects to explore the therapeutic value of computer usage. When one's personal kingdom of competence and control is shrinking, the power of a computer can be liberating. In a 1996 study (Sherer) nursing home residents and day care participants were divided into a research group and a control group. The group that used the personal computer increased scores in self-esteem and life satisfaction.

In a contrasting review of computer-mediated self-help groups for older women (Kaye, 1997), observers found a broad array of online forums: Widowed World, Over Fifty and Having Fun, Depression Mutual Support, and many other similar choices. But the average older woman in the community lacked the equipment and the training to take advantage of technology. Local support groups continued to meet face to face. They made no organized attempt to obtain computers by either donation or subsidy.

David Lansdale, a geriatrics expert from Stanford University, believes every nursing home should be equipped with communal e-mail and internet access (1999). It is an elixir for elders who are lonely, bored, helpless, and mentally declining. After his 12-week course of instruction, residents testify that the Internet has become a new window to life.

Now many assisted living and nursing care facilities are setting up computer labs (Daniel, 1998). Equipment is donated by corporations or individuals who are upgrading their own systems. Most of the cost is due to dedicated space and salary for an on-site technician (often part-time). A cadre of high school students and other volunteers train the residents. Once a core of residents has conquered the recycled computers, they become peer teachers. Enthusiasm goes up each time a grandchild is contacted by e-mail.

Microsoft Senior Initiative aims at bridging digital and generational divides by providing access to PC training and tools. It is a resource for seniors, their families, and communities. In 1999 they established a technology award for older adults. Another well-know organization, Senior Net, helps set up learning labs if facilities are willing to donate space. The group has learning centers in almost every state. In 1998 Senior Explorer Network was founded. It claims to be "a virtual meeting place where seniors can partake in many activities without being bothered with some of the complexities inherent in the internet" (Etchegoyen, 2000).

PREDICTORS OF COMPUTER USE BY THE AGED

Some of the oldest generation will be enthusiastic about learning computers because they want to keep up with cyber-savvy children and grandchildren. Others are inhibited and afraid to be seen as incompetent. There are ways to predict their accomplishment. What previous skills have they already mastered?

- Use of the touchtone phone shows they can listen and remember a list of menu choices. They can see and press numbers on a keypad (probably enlarged). They can wait patiently on Hold.
- Use of a typewriter, cash register, or other keyboard shows dexterity and acumen.
- Use of automated teller machines shows they have a high level of trust in automated systems. They like services that are available at

any time and practically anywhere. They have no overblown fear of robbers at remote, outdoor locations.

- Use of Web TV (or other internet appliance) shows they have learned to use the wireless keyboard, to scroll, to click, to browse the Internet, to send and receive e-mail. They may have tried interactive features like quiz shows. Dreyfuss (2000) reports high popularity of Web TV with noncomputer-users.

BARRIERS

The oldest generation will be the least likely to try computers for a variety of reasons, some of which are based on experience, some on hearsay evidence, and some on inadequate knowledge. Consider the following barriers and the ways they might be overcome:

1.   Unfamiliarity. People are easily intimidated by a new machine. When the video cassette recorder was first marketed late night comics had a heyday. The butt of all jokes was the guy who couldn't even program a VCR. Beyond the fear of breaking the computer is the fear of losing data when there are other users. Frequency of use can overcome this problem. The old gentleman who watches an aide click in his menu choices every day will soon want to point and click himself.

2.   Sensory deficits. Because so much reading is involved, vision is a key issue. Web TV puts large, readable type on the screen. But PC's can change font (letter) size, magnify parts, or change background color or texture to make the screen more readable. Special lighting can reduce glare, and glasses can be made for the proper focal distance.

3.   Kinesthesia. This movement and pressure sense is important too. Learners are embarrassed when random movements bring up a response and intentional movements don't register. Touch, pressure, and dexterity are needed to handle keyboard and mouse. Variations on the latter are the IntelliMouse, track balls, and such, but they become familiar with use. Only the mini-mouse on a portable computer is unlikely to suit seniors.

4.   Decline in problem-solving ability (Seigler, 1980). While learning is the acquisition of skills, problem solving means using those

skills to make choices. Because the computer is designed to do many jobs, it requires more flexibility and analysis than operating the largely mechanical, single-purpose machines of the industrial age. The same computer can be a calculator, a typewriter, a search and scan tool, and more. Memorizing commands and layout is futile because technology and software change so rapidly.

5.   Perceptual "freeze." Like students in a test situation, elders are subject to perceptual freeze. They make a hasty assumption and hang on to it rigidly. They fail to see alternate paths, broader interpretations, or narrower categories. Skilled computer users are flexible, make educated guesses, and don't dwell on errors. For the elderly, "user friendly" means more commonality in procedures, functions, menus, and terminology. Responding to a dialog box, for instance, requires understanding the "language." Elders know the computer has a more reliable memory than they and feel relieved not to have to memorize control key combinations.

6.   Lack of education and training. While women may have had experience typing, many men have never used a keyboard. Unless voice-recognition machines are available, the hunt and peck system of input is workable. There is a special ego-booster, too, in the spelling and grammar checks. An e-mail message sent to a grandchild will not have any telltale errors.

7.   Lack of trust. Many elderly are wary and fear that one click could commit them to a financial burden. In June 2000 President Clinton signed the E-Sign Act which makes digital signatures legal for contracts, transactions, and records. Internet users can buy a car, get life insurance, or take out a mortgage without the need to sign and mail documents (Einstein, 2000). Likewise, corporations can computerize entirely the process of signing contracts to buy and sell products and services. In a poll of over 1000 elderly, the American Association of Retired Persons (2000) found that fully 70% feel "insecure" in their current computer skills. Only 8% rated themselves "expert." A substantial number were unwilling or unable to spend money to maintain or upgrade their systems. Eighty percent were concerned about privacy of information. They object to having their Internet activity tracked without permission. Fortunately, the E-Sign Act has some protective elements: consumers will not be required to use or accept digital signatures if they prefer paper.

8.   Frustration and embarrassment. When something goes wrong like a screen freezing or an error message, the learner feels guilty.

"You have performed an illegal procedure" is intimidating vocabulary. So there should be an on-site helper available whenever the computer room is open. The aging novice feels embarrassed to ask for help unless the trainers share some of their own "goofs." The more frequently the learner works with the system, the more quickly he/she can become a peer trainer and the fewer times mishaps are likely to occur. When instruction focuses on e-mail, games, or favorite places the learners experience immediate, pleasurable feedback and focus on the "how to's."

BENEFITS

Perhaps the oldest generation has the most to gain from computers. With a PC they can transcend time and space even though memory and mobility lapse. The Internet can bring the world into any room and research the past for facts and meaning. Elders can order groceries or research the family tree. Consider the following benefits against the alarmist tales of viruses, cybertheft, and exploitation.

Computers fill up time enjoyably.   Computer screens are more engaging and interactive than television. While habitual soap opera viewers might disagree about the passivity of TV, random viewers find the plots to be disconnected and the emotions overblown. Every move of a cursor does something and the screen can carry several diversions at once. Each menu choice gives the user a sense of power, just like pushing a call button and finding a nurse or an airline attendant at your side. Card players who can't find a partner for bridge can play with people all across the Internet. Yahoo games, for instance, include chess, checkers, backgammon, go, dominoes, majong, blackjack, cribbage, hearts, and some solitaire games, along with computer auto racing, baseball, and golf.

Computers provide socialization.   In a full month study of 3533 adults (Jesdanun, 2000) it was found that friends and relatives communicated more frequently because of the Internet. The e-mail exchanges were bits of news, jokes, and everyday conversations. Where handwritten letters had had an advantage of being read and reread and shown to friends, e-mails can be printed out and photographs (digitized) attached. Letters still tend to be more thoughtful and serious, perhaps because the act of writing gives time to reflect. This study showed that deeply emotional topics were avoided online. Women were more likely than men to credit the Internet for improving family ties.

Chat rooms allow seniors to cross age barriers to make new friends. Anonymity can be dangerous for the gullible, but for elders it can be an escape from a decrepit appearance that masks the inner spirit. Chat rooms cannot replace face-to-face communication, but they can be simpler, less frustrating, and less stressful. At best, they can provide socialization as the senior always wished it might be . . . courteous, consoling, intimate, and ageless.

Computers provide mental stimulation. Youngsters have proven that computers can rivet attention and increase its span. So game-playing is a good way to start teaching elders. Moving from action-reaction sequences to more conventional card games stretches the memory to cover an increasing sequence of action. Reading fiction (e-books) stretches memory of people, places, and plot. It also stimulates analysis of human motives. Reading nonfiction e-books can lead to the highest levels of reasoning as can participation in news groups or finance clubs.

Computers promote mental health. Beyond chat rooms there are a broad range of support and self-help groups on the Internet. A fine example is the webwhispers organization founded by "Dutch" Helms (2000). It is a support group and information site for people with cancer of the larynx. Comprised of 82 pages and 329 graphics on its own independent server, it provides factual and referral information that is comprehensive, accurate, and up-to-date. Over 3000 visitors per month can also get real time assistance via e-mail. The site has been rated as "outstanding" by Medindex, Excite At Home, Sympatico, and the American Academy of Otolaryngology, Head, and Neck Surgery. Typical of the grassroots vigor of computer-literate seniors, volunteers from WebWhispers fully designed, built, and published a website for the traditional International Association of Larynectomees (IAL).

So many adult health problems are chronic, ongoing, and irreversible that keeping up morale is as important as managing symptoms.

An inspiring comment comes from Steve Mallory, a contributing writer for the *Stroke Connection*. When asked if he felt disabled, he replied "Not on the computer." His regular column "Stroke on the Web" links families to stroke information and resources, from scientific abstracts to survivors' homepages. Support groups for specific ailments allow patients to adjust and assimilate to new conditions with a sympathetic group of survivors. It spares friends and family some of the necessary venting and rehearsal prior to taking on a new role. The Princeton Survey Research Association (Jesdanun, 2000) found that women were more likely than men to seek health and religious information online. Rather than experiencing isolation they found like-minded friends.

Some health care providers are offering mental health and substance abuse counseling on the Internet. An interactive Web site gives assistance on stress, depression, smoking cessation, nutrition, personal growth, and behavior topics. Originally designed for working adults, the program content and methodology are well-known features in the cyberworld.

Computers provide health information.   At the turn of the century 77 million people had gone to the Internet for health information (Gearon, 2000). Among them were seniors trying to stay on top of medical developments affecting themselves and their loved ones. Since managed care systems tend to reduce each patient's time with doctors, computers offer a valuable way to increase understanding. There are 20,000 Web sites devoted to health care with as many more related sites (dealing with diet, alternative medicine, etc.). Only a few sites have been checked and approved by experts, as there is no central authority monitoring the accuracy and honesty of Web pages. Dot coms may mix editorial copy with advertisements. The pages run by government agencies or nonprofit groups may lack the pizzazz of .com pages, but may inform as reliably as a medical library. Individuals who surf these sources are on the way to self-efficacy.

When the patient uses interactive sites his/her privacy may be compromised. Although surfing the Internet has some risk, seniors have the experience to sniff out scams. They know that vague directions for use, emotional language, and sunny promises of cures can signal quackery. They choose National Institutes of Health sites like

PubMed or state-sponsored sites like New York's NOAH. They gather information as an adjunct to, not a substitute for, physician care.

EXERCISES

1. Explore the following three websites. What do they offer? How do they help seniors live a rational life, a sociable life, or a more profitable life? Add three websites that suit particular hobbies seniors might have.
    a. www.seniorexplorer.com
    b. www.eldertek.com
    c. www.seniornet.org

2. Here is a list of websites useful for managing health and general welfare:

www.alfa.org	Assisted Living Federation
www.sleepfoundation.org	
www.healthdesign.org	
www.careguide.net	
www.caregiver.org	
www.diabetes.org	
www.alz.org	Alzheimer's Disease
www.amhrt.org	American Heart Association
www.cancer.org	
www.aarp.org/griefandloss	
www.aarp.org/cyber/sitealph.htm	AARP guide to internet
www.nlm.nih.gov	National Library of Medicine
www.nimh.nih.gov	National Institute of Mental Health

    Visit these sites and rank them on a scale of one to ten for "user friendliness."

REFERENCES

American Association of Retired Persons (2000, March). National survey on consumer preparedness and E-commerce (Executive Summary). Washington, DC: author. Available at http://research.aarp.org/consumer/ecommerce_l.html [2000, August 1].

Daniel, A. (1998). Seniors in cyberspace. *Contemporary Long Term Care*, *32*, 89–91.

Dreyfuss, J. (2000). I want my WebTV. *Modern Maturity*, *43*, 90–91.

Einstein, D. (2000, June 30) Clinton signs Digital Signature Act. Forbes [Online]. Available at: http://www.forbes.com/ [2000, July 1].

Etchegoyen, C. (2000). What is the senior explorer network? [Online]. Webmaster. Available at: http://www.seniorexplorer.com/ [2000, July 10].

Gearon, C. (2000). Going online for health. *AARP Bulletin*, *41*(5), 14–16.

Helms, D. (2000, Apr 14). Laryngeal cancer information website. [Online] Webmaster. Available at: http://www.webwhispers.org./pages/basic.htm [2000, June 5].

Jesdanun, A. (2000, May 11). Friends and family connect more using the net. *San Francisco Examiner*, p. 12.

Kaye, L. (1997). *Self-help support groups for older women*. Washington, DC: Taylor & Francis.

Lansdale, D. (1999, Nov.). Internet gives the elderly a link to life. Paper presented at Gerontological Society of America, San Diego, CA.

McConnaughey, J. (1998). Falling through the net II: New data on the digital divide. Washington, DC: National Telecommunications and Information Administration. Available at http://www.ntiadoc.gov/ntiahome/net2/falling.html [2000, July 20].

Romich, B. (2000). *The road to funding*. Wooster, OH: Prentke Romich.

Seigler, I. (1980). The psychology of adult development and aging. In E. Busse & D. Blazer (Eds.), *Handbook of geriatric psychiatry*. New York: Van Nostrand Reinhold.

Sherer, L. M. (1996). The impact of using personal computers on the lives of nursing home residents. *Physical and Occupational Therapy in Geriatrics*, *14*(2), 13–28.

10

Preserving Morale

A variety of psychological tests and sociological surveys have tried to determine the happiness of individuals. Government authorities often try to evaluate the service programs they offer older people in terms of how they affect morale. When such tests concentrate on participation they may be measuring simply extroversion and introversion. Since those personality attributes remain relatively stable through life, they tell nothing about an individual's sense of satisfaction with life at any one point in time.

It is too simplistic to assume that the outwardly warm, friendly, easygoing person must feel good inside, and that the aloof, laconic type is miserable. The cheerful backslapper may be secretly depressed and neurotic, and the recluse may lead a life of quiet contentment. Further, neither individual is uncommunicative when all forms of communication are considered—listening, reading, and writing, as well as talking. Interactions need not be frequent to be meaningful and satisfying.

HAPPINESS IS . . . A PERSONAL PERCEPTION

In the late 1960s, the University of Chicago (Neugarten, 1968) did an extensive study of life-satisfaction, social role activity, and personality patterns of healthy persons aged 70 to 79. Of the eight personality patterns delineated, only two types rated low on life satisfaction. They were the unintegrated personalities with gross defects in psychologic function and an apathetic group with low activity ratings. In the latter, were a man who let his wife do his talking for him and a woman dedicated solely to meeting her physical needs. The scarcity of communication forms was notable even without overwhelming biologic accidents like stroke or cancer. These people had simply not chosen to be part of the social circle of communication.

Later studies used the Life Satisfaction Rating Scale developed by Neugarten or ratings on the Philadelphia Geriatric Center Morale Scale. They showed that what makes up happiness is a personal matter, but there are factors almost everyone desires—good health, adequate money, and someone to be with and confide in.

Of the other factors involved in happiness—children, owning a home, job success, and so forth—both young and old responders gave them widely different ratings. For the elderly group, Siebert and Mutran (1999) found that the role of "friend" was the strongest predictor of life satisfaction—stronger than income or marital status.

In a thoughtful review of the difficulties in measuring quality of life Lawton (1997) argues that health cannot be included in a single-score test. Topics like medical outcomes, functional health, and acute and chronic physical illness are best addressed in separate surveys. Generally there is a higher correlation between self-reported health and morale than between objective health and morale.

Rather than struggling to reach a single measure Lawton suggests that quality of life be assessed in four domains. The objective, social-normative component can be judged by outsiders. It includes residential environment (security, comfort . . .) and behavioral competence (in self-chosen activities). The subjective, intrapersonal domains are perceived quality of everyday life and general psychological well-being.

Assessing life satisfaction is complex because subjective perception colors all self-reports. Morale is more closely related to perceptions of self and circumstances than to objective facts and circumstances. While practitioners often cannot change the actual physical detriments and the irrevocable losses that older persons have suffered, they can help older persons with the negative and demoralizing perceptions of those decrements and losses.

In a study of community-based elderly Mannell (1993) found high life satisfaction in persons who had high-investment activities. Passive leisure activities lacked flow and commitment. But freely chosen activities that challenged skills and required an investment of effort resulted in very positive feelings.

KEEPING ATTITUDES FLEXIBLE

Skinner and Vaughan (1983) decry the fact that many of the attitudes held by the elderly militate against their happiness. Yet these same attitudes were beneficial at earlier stages and were instrumentally rewarded by society. For instance, being "thrifty" at age 17 becomes "stinginess" at 71, or being "sober-minded" at 25 becomes "grouchiness" at 75. What was trained as socially desirable behavior becomes a lifelong habit, even when it no longer suits the living conditions and physical capabilities of the aged individual.

Consider the mental activity called rationalizing and how it is perceived over time. The young woman who drops out of college explains that she does not like her instructors or does not want to live so far away from her boyfriend. Here the meaning of rationalize is "to invent plausible explanations for acts that are actually based on other causes, possibly unconscious." Perhaps she really has an overwhelming fear of failing. Do-gooders and go-getters consider "rationalizing" a pejorative term.

Consider the aged professor who is invited to speak at the national convention of a 50,000-member professional organization. He knows that his memory will not allow him to speak without notes. He knows that his vision problem and the kind of lighting in vast halls will not allow him to see his notes or make eye contact with his audience. He knows none of his cohorts will be going and he forgets the names of younger colleagues. He knows he will have trouble finding his way around different buildings and hotels. He graciously declines the invitation. He is operating under another definition of rationalize, that is, "to act in conformance with reason."

But the old man is angry, depressed, and disgusted with his body and its faltering senses and systems. He is ashamed, because he still carries the negative connotations of rationalizing. He sees his current behavior not as a sign of wisdom and reason, but as a weakness. The do-or-die attitude that helped him build his career makes him feel defeated at the time of relinquishing that career. Logically, he knows he made the right decision, but he remains in a "blue funk" for days.

The dogged determination that helps the young achieve in everything from athletics to academics creates discontent in the old. And facing inevitable and irreversible changes with discontent is hardly a just reward for a life of hard work and perseverance. Rigid attitudes hurt.

COGNITIVE RESTRUCTURING

Negative thinking can be combated with cognitive restructuring. The process involves changing the negative messages you send to yourself into more realistic positive ones. Highly charged emotions distorted the perceptions on which the first message was based so it takes conscious effort to see positive factors in the situation. For example, an Olympic skier notices that his major competitor skies the slalom in 9.6 minutes. Instead of worrying, "I can't beat that time," the skier uses cognitive restructuring to tell himself, "That time means the course must be in great shape. Now I can do it, too."

The oldster faced with a prohibition against caffeine has to restructure "I can't start the day without my coffee," into "I'm so glad I got a chance to 'scotch' those Brazilians! When I think what I've paid for coffee and would have to pay now! Why I could have bought my own plantation. Besides, I feel better."

A reminiscing discussion group can practice cognitive restructuring by telling about past events that started out bad but were turned to good effect. Rigidity can decline when past experiences of getting "a lemon and turning it into lemonade" are remembered and relived.

Cousins (1991), former editor of the Saturday Review, combatted his own death sentence with positive thinking. He recommended that health professionals use cognitive restructuring in their messages to severely ill patients:

> Good doctors propose a partnership. They describe what medical science has to offer . . . and what the patient has to offer. . . . For a patient to be told that two of every five persons with a certain illness do not last out the year is not as useful or as motivating as to be told that three of five patients overcome their illness.

IMAGING

The process of visualizing a desired behavior or response is called "imaging." It is a mental rehearsal of an action in which the muscles are programmed for peak efficiency. In terms of sports, a golf pro says, "I never hit a shot, not even in practice, without having a sharp, in-focus picture of it in my head." In terms of rehabilitation, the oldster can think through the exercise for a weakened arm or leg before enacting it.

Occupational therapists encourage the disabled person to approach a household task, like slicing onions, by visualizing. Comments such as "Let's plan it out first. Is the board secure? How will you have to position the knife? Which way will the slices fall?" produce pictures in the mind of the activity before it occurs so any corrective maneuvers can be mentally rehearsed. Nurses use imagery in providing health care (Balzer-Riley, 2000). They model positive self-talk as they perform procedures that may be uncomfortable or embarrassing.

Imaging positive results in communication activities is not as easy because of the two-way nature of the process. Although the other party cannot be controlled, sensitive reading of feedback can lead the speaker to send more appropriate messages. The oldster who bypasses criticizing, moralizing, and complaining to visitors usually gets more visitors. Skinner, a renowned psychologist, suggests "imaging" the final stage of life as simply another role to be played: "When played with skill the part of Old Person is marked by tranquility, wisdom, freedom, dignity and a sense of humor" (Skinner & Vaughan, 1983, p. 141).

INNOVATIVE APPROACHES

Old people are often accused of being stubborn or "set in their ways." They cannot handle the changes in their lives or meet new challenges unless they perceive reality, relationships, and alternatives. Perhaps rigidity of attitudes can be countered with exercise just as muscular rigidity is. If various mental sets are experienced and practiced the oldster can select which reactions and perceptions he/she wishes to live by.

A young recreation therapist reported on an innovation he developed for small discussion groups. He called it a "bingo" game:

1. Draw a large bingo card on the blackboard or flip chart.
2. Choose a single topic: cars, babies, voting, cotton candy, hospitals, and so forth.
3. Elicit from group members their reactions to the topic—at various stages in life:
   B: Beginning—reaction at *age 17* (e.g., loved cars, hated babies)
   I: In-between—reaction at *mid-life* (e.g., loved babies, hated hospitals)
   N: Now—reaction in *seventies* (e.g., cool on cars, warmer on hospitals)
4. Write down several of the reactions in the box spaces under each letter.
5. Elicit comments on what is a good attitude to take toward the topic and what is an opposite attitude. Emulate a business person's thinking—best-case, worst-case scenarios.
6. Write under *G* the *good attitudes*. Write under *O* the *opposite ones*, so people can remember and discuss them further.

A colleague working at a nursing home for long-term care used the same bingo scoreboard idea in a different way. She was working with new residents, trying to guide them into new friendships. Her goal was to pair up "buddies" who could assist in physical care and "confidantes" who could assist in mental and emotional care. She began by working on communication/conversation behaviors. Her "bingo" chart represented:

B: Brevity. Give examples of times you limited your talking so someone else could talk too.

I: Interest. How did you show interest in someone else's story?

N: Negotiation. Tell how you and your friends decide what to do on a shopping day. How did you "give and take" in making decisions in your family?

G: Gumption. How did you show gumption in taking care of yourself? What positive assertions did you make? How did you act differently to break up rigid habits or ideas?

O: Opting for humor. How can you make your mealtime companions chuckle? Tell a joke for today.

BUILDING MORALE WITH HOSPITALITY

During the last two decades there has been reassuring growth in the health communications field. Schools of nursing, allied health, and medicine are requiring their students to learn how to talk with their patients. Through role-playing and model interactions students become aware that patients are not simply samples of a disease, but total human beings.

Recently, hospitals began promoting humane care by providing training in common courtesies to all staff members. The hospital business has become increasingly competitive because of changes in insurance policies, dwindling government support, and the trend toward outpatient services. Friendliness became a way to attract health consumers just as airlines woo travelers by offering perks and friendly service.

Albert Einstein Medical Center in New York led the trend. After consulting with nine local hotel executives for advice in handling patients, they made changes, such as better food, easier-to-read name tags, more accessible information desks, and radios/TVs in rooms. The hospitality program set rules:

- Make eye contact.
- Introduce yourself.
- Call people by name.
- Explain what you are doing.

Courtesy and friendliness assuage the trauma of hospitalization for all patients, but they are a special boon for the elderly. Finally, the elderly can find the respectful treatment for which they have longed.

In a skilled nursing facilities similar programs train staff in listening, clarifying, reassuring, and supporting (Pilkington, 1993). After only 12 weeks nurses and aides improved communication skills significantly. Residents cared for by the experimental group showed increased life satisfaction by scoring higher on the Philadelphia Geriatric Moral Scale.

PRESERVING MORALE BY HONORING

In the discussion of motivation, Maslow's hierarchy was cited because it recognizes the strong need for ego gratification. With increasing age it is more difficult to maintain status and live up to a positive image of oneself.

In contrast, the distinguished writer, editor, critic, and poet Cowley (1980) writes of the vanity of the aged. He defines it as a craving to be loved or simply admired. Were he not an octagenarian, he might have used the more timely term "status" or "self-esteem." Regardless, he intends to erase the pejorative connotations of vanity:

> The vanity of older people is easy to explain and to condone. With less to look forward to, they yearn for recognition of what they have been: the reigning beauty, the athlete, the soldier, the scholar. Often the yearning to be recognized appears in conversation as an innocent boast . . . to be admired and praised, especially by the young, is an autumnal pleasure enjoyed by the lucky ones. . . . That search for honors is a harmless passion. Honors cost little. Why shouldn't the very old have more than their share of them?

Fortunately, many ordinary oldsters can find respect and recognition within their own family and social circle. Without national notoriety, great power, or wealth, they appreciate the honors accorded for wedding anniversaries and birthdays. In long-term care facilities, where former status is blurred, there is still pleasure in celebrating one more year. Why, then, do institutions celebrate that annual birthday with a sweet, a song, and, perhaps, a gift? That is the same kind of celebration a child gets! It does not meet the emotional needs of the elderly, nor does it enhance their self-concept. It does not stimulate the rehabilitation of the ill or disabled.

A well thought out, convincingly delivered speech of tribute is a more professional response. Whether it is composed by the activities director of a senior center, the recreation therapist at a nursing home, or by a colleague, club chairperson, or family member, it enhances the oldster's relationship to the audience and his/her own self-esteem. A little artistic, rhetorical skill can make the honoree, if not immortal, at least memorable in some way. Adding mythic analogies makes a larger than life impression, such as the following:

- "Aunt Jane, the Aries who became a social lion."
- "A former teacher, Mr. X., could be called the Socrates of Small Town, USA."

- "His childhood name 'Tiny Mite' turned out to be Dynamite when he enlisted in the Marines."
- "Grandma is the white dove of Peace."
- "Mrs. X likes to be called an American Beauty Rose, but she started out as Armenian Beauty Rose."

For a very special occasion a human services trainee composed the following tribute to her father-in-law:

> I would like to share with you some thoughts about my father-in-law, James Angelo. Like the patriarch of an old European family, Jim counts hundreds of people as his children. For years, he has modeled his life on Saint Joseph—the hard working carpenter, husband to Mary. Jim is not only Dad to his two sons Jim Jr. and Tom; he is also "Dad" to his 100 employees at the Manor Nursing Home, the 150 employees at the Oakdale Nursing Home, and the 65 employees at Parkland.
>
> He is a man who began life in poverty, the fourth of twelve Italian-American children. He worked his way to owning three nursing homes. He runs the business like a father caring for a large family.
>
> Sunday is the day to follow in Dad's footsteps, because you can see Saint Joseph most clearly. He and his wife drive to his childhood church, to attend mass and light a devotional candle. Later in the morning, he visits the nursing home to see "his girls" and visit the patients. By one o'clock, he will be back home fixing spaghetti sauce and meatballs for the family (in many "old country" homes, the sauce "soogoo" is the responsibility of the patriarch).
>
> Dad spends Sunday afternoon working in the woodshop or the garden. He has become an expert at both hobbies. By four o'clock, however, he will be clean and dressed, ready for the family to arrive. Two sons and daughters-in-law, grandchildren, nieces, grandnieces, and whoever else is in town will come by for drinks, food and talk, until the gracious host dozes off in his chair.
>
> Dad's is a simple life—steady work, clean living, and devotion to the human family. His caring for others is a natural outgrowth of his faith in God. Today I toast his 75 years and wish him 75 more!

Respect and the Self-Fulfilling Prophecy

Distinguished sociologist Palmore spent his sabbatical year at the Tokyo Institute of Gerontology investigating the traditional pattern

of Eastern ancestor respect under the impact of modern industrialization. Among his cross-cultural insights was this:

> The very idea of a vertical society and of ancestor worship would seem
> alien, if not completely repugnant, to most Americans. Yet, . . . that
> respect for the aged is the key element which can maintain the status
> and integration of the aged in the family life and economic life of
> modern society. (Palmore, 1975)

Certainly older adults want to be useful, to be part of the mainstream. As they complete their own life cycle they try to build strength
in the next generation. The term generativity was coined by Erik
Erikson, an expert in human development (Erikson, Erikson, &
Kivnick, 1992). He noted that positive identity came from cultivating
the next generation within the family and within the community.

The very first paragraph of this book stated that our current society
stops expecting and stops receiving meaningful contributions from
the elderly. Is it not possible that the trend can be reversed? Receiving
respect is a strong motivation for behavior worthy of respect.

The German philosopher, Goethe, after many years of studying
the human condition, concluded, "Treat people as if they were what
they ought to be and you help them to become what they are capable
of being."

EXERCISES

1. Write a draft about some older person's life-memories of the
   First World War, for instance. Then have other students in the
   class interview you about that person. To what extent did their
   probing make you provide additional information or help you
   gain new insights.
2. Read the interview form below to help prepare a speech of
   introduction. Fill in the identification and pleasurable activities
   parts for yourself. Prepare a speech introducing yourself to
   your classmates.
3. To make your self-identification more graphic, interesting, and
   memorable, try aligning your personality characteristics with
   those of an animal, a famous person in history, a TV celebrity,

etc. Write a 100-word paragraph introducing yourself in this less ordinary way.

Interview for Information Leading to a Speech of Introduction/Tribute

Identification

1. What is your name?
2. Does it have a special meaning? (foreign, astrological sign, occupation, etc.)
3. What is your nickname?
4. Why do people call you that?
5. How do other people characterize you?

Gainful preoccupations

1. What kind of work do you do/have you done?
2. Just what does that entail?
3. Can you explain the big picture?
4. What was the most crucial event in your career?

Activities for pleasure

1. What are your hobbies?
2. Which is most fascinating?
3. Exactly what is involved?
4. What do others say about it (prizes, recognition, humor)?
5. What other things give you pleasure?
6. What was your most significant contribution (to your family, church, community)?
7. How do you want to be remembered?

4. Visit an older person and fill out the interview for information leading to a speech of introduction/tribute. Prepare a speech for either purpose to present to your classmates. Study the Evaluation Form that follows as you prepare. Those items represent the things people notice when you make an address.
5. Deliver the speech. Have someone rank you on the Speech Evaluation Form.

Speech Evaluation Form

Speaker: ———————————— date: ————————————

Title of speech: ——————————————————————————

Evaluate the speech according to the scale: 1 = low . . . 5 = high

Physical aspects

Enthusiasm	1	2	3	4	5
Visual directness	1	2	3	4	5
Posture	1	2	3	4	5
Movement	1	2	3	4	5
Gestures	1	2	3	4	5
Facial expression	1	2	3	4	5
Uses of the voice	1	2	3	4	5
Pace, rate of speaking	1	2	3	4	5
Pronunciation, articulation	1	2	3	4	5

Speech content

Attention-getting opener	1	2	3	4	5
Clear identification	1	2	3	4	5
Description of qualities	1	2	3	4	5
Clarity of details and explanations	1	2	3	4	5
Sufficient examples	1	2	3	4	5
Concluding tribute	1	2	3	4	5

REFERENCES

Balzer-Riley, J. (2000). *Communication in nursing* (4th ed.). St. Louis, MO: Mosby.

Cousins, N. (1991). *The anatomy of an illness as perceived by the patient.* New York: Bantam.

Cowley, M. (1980). *The view from eighty.* New York: Viking Penguin.

Erikson, E., Erikson, J., & Kivnick, H. (1992). *Vital involvement in old age.* New York: Norton.

Lawton, M. P. (1997). Measures of quality of life and subjective well-being. *Generations, 21,* 45–48.

Mannell, R. (1993). High-investment activity and life satisfaction among older adults: committed, serious leisure, and flow activities. In J. Kelly (Ed.), *Activity and aging.* Newbury Park, CA: Sage.

Neugarten, B. (1968). Developmental perspectives. *Psychiatric Research Reports. American Psychiatric Association, 23,* 42–48.

Palmore, E. (1975). *The honorable elders.* Durham, NC: Duke University Press.

Pilkington, W. (1993). Effects of a communication program on nursing home staff's communication skills and residents' levels of life satisfaction. Unpublished doctoral dissertation. St. John's University, New York.

Siebert, D., & Mutran, E. (1999). Friendship and social support: The importance of role identity to aging adults. *Social Work, 44,* 522–534.

Skinner, B. F., & Vaughan, M. E. (1983). *Enjoy old age: A program of self-management.* New York: W. W. Norton.

Index